To Brenda & Richard.

I am so
glad  wed
you

with love

Steven

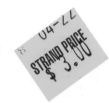

Love Again, Live Again

Steven Morganstern, M.D.
Allen Abrahams, Ph.D.

A James Peter Book
James Peter Associates, Inc.

PRENTICE HALL
Englewood Cliffs, New Jersey 07632

Prentice-Hall International (UK) Limited, *London*
Prentice-Hall of Australia Pty. Limited, *Sydney*
Prentice-Hall Canada, Inc., *Toronto*
Prentice-Hall Hispanoamericana, S.A., *Mexico*
Prentice-Hall of India Private Limited, *New Delhi*
Prentice-Hall of Japan, Inc., *Tokyo*
Simon & Schuster Asia Pte. Ltd., *Singapore*
Editora Prentice-Hall do Brasil, Ltda., *Rio de Janeiro*

© 1988 *by*

PRENTICE-HALL, INC.

Englewood Cliffs, NJ

10 9 8 7 6 5 4 3 2 1

Printed in the United States of America

Library of Congress Cataloging-in-Publication Data
Morganstern, Steven.
    Love again, live again / Steven Morganstern, Allen
Abrahams.
        p.   cm.
    "A James Peter book."
    Includes index.
    ISBN 0-13-540758-3
    1. Impotence—Popular works. I. Abrahams. Allen E. II.
Title.
RC889.M758 1988   88-22526
616.6'92—dc 19   CIP

ISBN 0-13-540758-3

PRENTICE HALL
BUSINESS & PROFESSIONAL DIVISION
A division of Simon & Schuster
Englewood Cliffs, New Jersey 07632

Dedication

To Barbra, Evan, and Brad, and in memory of Joel.

--S.M.

Acknowledgments

A book of this nature could not have been written without the input of many individuals. We are grateful for background provided on the dimensions of the impotence problem by F. Brantley Scott, M.D., Baylor College of Medicine, and William L. Furlow, M.D., formerly of the Mayo Clinic and now with The Center for Urological Treatment and Research, Nashville.

Jerry L. Freeman, American Diabetes Association, Georgia Affiliate, Inc., provided useful information on the important impotence-diabetes link. Robert L. Thompson, Ph.D., Hunter College, City University of New York, provided interesting background on psychological factors. Important contributions were also made by the staffs of the Atlanta Center for Male Sexual Dysfunction and the Diabetes Treatment Centers of America.

We were greatly assisted in the preparation of the final manuscript by our editors, Ellen Lohsen and Kathryn Dix. Our agent, Herbert F. Holtje, James Peter Associates, Inc., provided invaluable assistance, especially with respect to the basic concept and approach employed in the preparation of the book. We are also grateful for the encouragement of Lee Walburn, *Atlanta Magazine*, and the valuable assistance of Barbra Morganstern and Elaine Abrahams. Special thanks are due for the important insights offered by Jesse and Susan French, R. Russ and Junell L. Homer, and Jack Nichols.

Finally, the book would not have been possible without the very meaningful observations of countless former patients.

About the authors

*D*r. *Steven Morganstern* is a prominent urologist in private medical practice in Atlanta, Georgia. At the Morganstern Urology Clinic, Atlanta, Dr. Morganstern specializes in the diagnosis and treatment of impotence and other forms of male sexual dysfunction. In the course of his practice, he has implanted over 1,200 inflatable penile implants in impotent patients. Dr. Morganstern serves as Director of the Atlanta Center for Male Sexual Dysfunction and Coordinator of Urologic Services for Diabetes Treatment Centers, Atlanta Georgia. In addition, Dr. Morganstern is actively engaged in research and professional and public education in the area of male sexual dysfunction. His research activities have included pioneering efforts in the fields of penile injection therapy and penile implants. Educational activities have included frequent lectures to physicians and other medical professionals on techniques for the treatment of male sexual dysfunction and extensive radio, television, and lecture activities directed toward the general public. His efforts resulted in the establishment of the first impotence support group in the Atlanta area. Dr. Morganstern is an honors graduate of the University of

Missouri School of Medicine. His past professional connections include the Ellis Fischel State Cancer Center, Columbia, Missouri; Shaare Zedek Hospital, Jerusalem, Israel; Long Island Jewish Hospital; and the University of North Carolina, Chapel Hill.

Allen Abrahams, Ph.D., is a writer, consultant, and educator with a strong background in medical, pharmaceutical, scientific, and technological subjects. His professional activities have included many projects on behalf of pharmaceutical, chemical, and scientific equipment manufacturers in connection with applied medical technology and other medically related subjects. Dr. Abrahams holds a B.S. degree in chemical engineering from the University of Maryland, a M.S. in industrial engineering from the Stevens Institute of Technology, and a Ph.D. in economics from the New York University, Graduate School of Business Administration. Dr. Abrahams has lectured on a worldwide basis before university, business, professional, and consumer groups. He is a former senior member of the faculty of the Polytechnic University, New York.

Foreword

"The course of true love never did run smooth."
-- Shakespeare

Some couples are finding that the problem is not "loving" but "making love." There are perhaps hundreds of thousands of loving couples who are not sharing a physical relationship. There are as many single men who avoid any kind of relationship because they are physically unable to be sexually intimate.

The problem is impotence and the estimated ten million American men who suffer from it cannot enjoy normal intercourse. They simply can't.

Whether impotence is caused by a physical illness such as diabetes or high blood pressure, by a psychological problem, or by the pressure of life's complexities, it is a debilitating, devastating condition.

Someone wise once said the only time sex is overwhelmingly important is when it's bad. Such is the case with impotence.

Yet as important as impotence is, it still is not dealt with by many men or their partners.

A discussion of impotence still causes snickers. The very word sets off giggles, jokes, and laughter. Men seem compelled to tell you they never have that problem! Publicly, women seem to find the whole thing pretty amusing.

Privately, however, men and their partners suffer.

Impotence is simply the inability for a man to have an erection good enough to have sex.

Does that sentence embarrass you? You would not be alone if it does.

Words like erection, penis, and intercourse make most of us uncomfortable. That's one of the reasons men often don't seek help. It's part of the reason some couples pretend for years that there is no problem and instead choose to stop all sexual activity and avoid the embarrassment of sexual failure.

As a result, nobody talks and nobody learns.

That's also one of the reasons Dr. Steven Morganstern wrote *Love Again, Live Again*. He's seen more than 8,000 men who have come for help because of an impotence problem. He has heard the pain and felt the joy when impotence is resolved.

Which is why *Love Again, Live Again* is thirteen chapters of invaluable information.

If you have a problem, think you have a problem, worry about having a problem some day or, if your partner is a man with an impotence problem, *Love Again, Live Again* can be the first step.

You don't have to talk about you or someone you love. You don't have to say one word out loud.

You need only read and learn. And begin to understand. This is a very valuable private education.

I think that what you are going to find is relief.

First, you are not alone. It is estimated that one in every ten adult men is impotent all or most of the time.

Second, something can be done. Many men suffer from guilt and depression as a result of their impotence. They come to believe they are no longer real men.

Well, they are wrong. Impotence can be fixed and there are thousands of men across the country who are proof of this.

Take a close look at Chapter 5. It offers a simple questionnaire that gives you a chance to consider the source and severity of the impotence in the privacy of your home.

Maybe it will help you pick up the phone and make an appointment with a qualified doctor.

Often it's the relationship between doctor and patient that can make the difference in solving an impotence problem. *Love Again, Live Again* offers guidelines on what you should expect from a doctor who is diagnosing and treating impotence. It's the doctor's job to "relax and relate" to the person seeking help.

This is a good book packed with practical, up-to-date information. It walks you through the treatment process step-by-step. After reading it, there won't be any surprises for an impotent man. You'll have a good sense of all the options.

The one caveat in this good news story brings us back to relationships. Even if impotence is caused by a physical problem, a penile implant or hormone injections will not repair a damaged or broken relationship. Impotence treatment only restores the ability to have an erection, not the ability to communicate and maintain a loving relationship.

As with any problem, expect to do some mending. Both partners need to adjust to whatever solution they choose for solving an impotence problem.

But, the fact remains that no one has to live with an impotence problem anymore. There are answers. Let this book be your guide.

Joyce Brothers, Ph.D.

How this book
will help you —
and your partner

I t is always rewarding to hear from the partners of men who have been successfully treated for sexual dysfunction. Susan did more than just send a short note. Instead, she wrote a detailed history of her husband's impotence problem, including how it nearly destroyed their marriage. She was thankful for the joyous change that took place after her husband obtained suitable professional treatment. In her letter, Susan expressed the hope that her experiences would help other couples with similar problems. Near the beginning of her story, Susan recalled the following:

> One evening we met friends for dinner. With dinner, Jesse had several drinks. While we were driving home, Jesse asked me why I had remained faithful to him. He could not understand why I did not have a lover. "I can't be a real husband to you when I'm only half a man."

Jesse and Susan were married in 1968, just twelve days after Jesse's return from Vietnam. About five years later, their marriage was a shambles, and a twelve-year period of "heartache, anxiety and frustration" followed. In Susan's words:

> Gradually our lives became a turmoil of anger and hurt, misunderstanding and jealousy. Jesse became withdrawn and secretive. I became defensive and resentful. We seldom made love, and on the rare occasions when we did, it was totally unsuccessful — leaving us both empty and unfulfilled.

Regardless of all logic and constant reassurance, the typical impotence victim is convinced that he is somehow less than a man. "Being a man" in the sexual sense is important in our culture, and, for that matter, in virtually every culture. Despite frequent media ridicule of the excesses of "machismo," many American men, regardless of education, awareness, and sensitivity, equate successful sexual performance with maleness, self-worth, and the respect and even loyalty of their partners. Little can be done to convince them to the contrary. Fame, power, financial success, children, hobbies or even a Nobel prize provide little compensation.

Impotence is equally trying for the female partner. In a classic impotence pattern, Susan placed much of the blame on herself. She reasoned that she had become unattractive and, hence, undesirable to her husband. She had gained weight during the early years of their marriage, and she felt that perhaps this was the real cause of the trouble. Susan recalls feeling that her life was over: her children and work could not replace the void in her life.

Susan's and Jesse's troubles eventually resulted in a two-year separation, although later they managed to reconcile. The eight years that followed were characterized by endless visits to marriage counselors, sex therapists, and health professionals, all of whom concluded that Jesse's problem was psychological in nature. None provided a workable solution. One even advised Susan to "dump" her husband while she was still young enough to start over.

Eventually, Jesse discovered that he had diabetes, a common cause of impotence. Susan recalls their almost perverse joy the day they learned that the underlying cause of their trouble was a potentially dangerous disease, rather than an emotional failing on their part. The diabetes, fortunately, could be controlled by diet. In contrast, implant surgery by a urologist was the only possible solution for Jesse's impotence problem.

Four weeks after surgery, Susan and Jesse successfully reconsummated their marriage. The long nightmare finally ended on the very day of their eighteenth wedding anniversary. Writing three months later, Susan reported some interesting changes in their life: the tension was gone, the children seemed happier, she felt prettier and was actively trying to lose weight, a co-worker had commented to Jesse on how much easier he was to get along with.

The nightmare that Susan and Jesse suffered had a happy ending. Millions of others have not been so lucky. Given an aging American population, the indiscriminate prescription of drugs for conditions such as hypertension, and other factors, impotence and other forms of male sexual dysfunction may be an increasingly common affliction. Fortunately, after years of misunderstanding, the scientific community and the general public are finally coming to understand and accept the underlying physical causes of sexual dysfunction. The pace of medical research especially since 1980, has accelerated. For the first time, there is now real hope for the majority of impotence sufferers. Moreover, help is now well within the budgetary limitations of most individuals.

The major purpose of this book is to provide a systematic self-help guide for people like Susan and Jesse. The widely held belief that almost all impotence has a psychological origin has yielded to the recognition that in up to 70 percent of the cases impotence can be traced to one or more very real physical problems. This book, therefore, places major emphasis on physical causes and physical solutions.

This is not meant to lessen the role and importance of psychological factors as a cause of impotence, nor is it meant to downplay the important contributions that psychotherapists and sex therapists have made and will continue to make in the study of impotence. Such therapy, after all, was virtually all that was available during the many years in which the impotence problem was ignored by the medical establishment. However, therapy, while it may help deal with the emotional pain that accompanies impotence, cannot cure the condition if it is caused by a physical problem.

The first four chapters of this book provide useful and interesting background on the nature of the impotence problem including a description of how the male sexual mechanism should normally work, how it can malfunction, and the problems that can cause a malfunction. Chapters 5 and 6 will help you determine whether professional help is advisable, and how best to go about obtaining effective help.

Chapters 7 through 10 outline the various treatment possibilities now available, to help you choose the best treatment plan for your circumstances. You'll learn exactly what to expect with each type of treatment approach. Chapter 11 covers the ever-important question of how much the treatment will cost, and provides information about insurance and tax considerations. Chapter 12 deals with the prevention of impotence and how you can delay its onset if you are in a high-risk category. Chapter 12 also includes tips for avoiding "impotence fraud."

The final chapter is addressed to Susan and to every other woman who shares in her partner's anguish. The female partner plays an important role in the successful treatment of male sexual dysfunction. This final chapter offers practical suggestions and advice on how she can both assist her partner and at the same time cope with her own difficulties.

Steven Morganstern, M.D.
Allen Abrahams, Ph.D.

Contents

CHAPTER 1

Why impotence
is more than
a sexual problem

The word "impotent" is used in common speech to describe a person of either gender lacking in power, strength, or vigor. At times, the meaning is broadened to imply the notion of helplessness. The word "impotence," as we will be using it, describes a familiar male sexual problem: a man who suffers from impotence is in some way incapable of normal sexual performance. Burdened with this condition, an impotent man has trouble enough without being told, or made to feel, that he is helpless. Nevertheless, the word that describes his medical problem does carry negative connotations that challenge his very worth as a human being.

WHAT IS IMPOTENCE?

The word "impotence" is used very narrowly in this book to describe only a specific and usually medically treatable condition of a physical nature: the inability of a man to achieve and maintain an erection, adequate for vaginal penetration, to the mutual satisfaction of both parties. Impotence is completely unrelated to the character of the individual who suffers from this condition, and the sufferer must not try to take responsibility or "blame" for it.

Impotence occurs in all men at one time or another. If the condition is experienced on a regular and persistent basis, it is referred to as chronic impotence and represents a medical problem that should never be ignored.

When your car fails to start on a cold winter morning, you may become angry, and you may even blame yourself for not having had the car properly tuned in warmer weather, but to remedy the situation you seek a mechanical solution; you do not blame the car! Similarly, this book emphasizes the physical nature of impotence and other problems of male sexual dysfunction and gives you scientific methods of diagnosis and treatment.

It is not certain how many American males suffer from impotence and other forms of sexual dysfunction. Impotence is not a contagious disease, required by law to be reported to public health authorities. Impotence victims have generally been "in the closet," usually too embarrassed to discuss their problems, even with their own physicians. Until quite recently, most American medical schools have regarded human sexuality in general, and especially male sexual dysfunction, as a taboo subject. In the past, the occasional researcher expressing interest in the field has often been viewed suspiciously by professional colleagues.

When was the last time, during an annual physical examination, that your doctor asked if you were experiencing any form of sexual dysfunction? Your doctor has probably never asked you such a question, even though sexual dysfunction can also be symptomatic of several serious underlying diseases.

WHY POTENCY IS IMPORTANT

Impotence is admittedly an unpleasant condition, both for the victim and his partner, but it is seldom life threatening. People can live without sexual gratification. In fact, throughout history many men and women have taken vows of chastity, often for reasons of religious belief, and have still lived rich, fulfilling lives. Many people consider today's preoccupation with sex a failing of modern society and a cause of social ills. In addition, treatment for sexual dysfunction can be expensive, and in a world where many are hungry, is often considered a personal indulgence. Nonetheless, there are several critical reasons why impotence must be dealt with:

1. Impotence and some other dysfunctions can prevent a man from fathering children.

2. Impotence strains family relationships.

3. Successful sexual performance indicates good health.

4. Impotence affects a man's job performance.

5. Sexual dysfunction can be linked to antisocial behavior.

6. Impotence is often a symptom of a serious underlying disease.

The ability to have children

People have sex for procreational, recreational, and relational purposes. While some may deprecate the necessity of recreational sex in the family relationship, few fail to sympathize with the personal anguish of a financially secure and responsible young couple unable to have children. Widespread support appears to exist for the well-publicized "test tube" approaches used in recent years to help infertile couples achieve pregnancy.

Failure to have children because of impotence places a very special emotional burden on the man. It is difficult enough for a man to be denied the pleasure of sexual intercourse and to fail to perform adequately as a lover. But the failure to have children because of impotence often makes the man feel that he has failed in his basic biological role to propagate the species. A man unable to have children due to some other problem, such as inadequate sperm count, may feel a sense of failure as well, but his guilt and self-loathing are inherently less than those of the man unable even to perform the act of sexual intercourse.

Treatment of impotence in childless couples can have very gratifying results. For example, consider the case of an impotent, twenty-five-year-old, married patient who had suffered from diabetes since childhood. Because of religious beliefs, artificial insemination was not an option for him and his wife. Anguished and suicidal, he had already separated from his wife. Successful treatment included the implantation of an inflatable penile device. One year later, the man and his wife reconciled, and now they are the very happy parents of a baby girl.

It is important to understand that there is no special connection between impotence and male sterility. A male with an inadequate sperm count may be perfectly capable of engaging in normal intercourse. This, of course, is commonly the case with a man who has had a vasectomy. An impotent male, however, may have a normal sperm count. He may be *able* to father a child. This could be accomplished if the man was able to successfully masturbate to ejaculation, despite his inability to achieve an adequate erection for intercourse. The resulting ejaculate can be artificially inseminated into the female partner. This approach, however, is heroic in nature, potentially expensive, has esthetic and psychological limitations, and may be unacceptable because of a patient's religious beliefs.

Impotence is not the only condition in which male sexual dysfunction results in the inability to have children. Successful impregnation is obviously a problem in the case of premature ejaculation and the condition known as retrograde ejaculation. In Peyronie's disease, the presence of scar tissue in the penis results in a bent erection, causing difficulty in achieving vaginal penetration and sometimes severe pain to both parties during intercourse. Other physical problems can make intercourse virtually impossible. Louis XVI of France, for many years, was unable to achieve penetration during intercourse with his wife, the notable Marie Antoinette, because of an exceptionally tight foreskin which prevented erection. The condition was surgically corrected, and the couple subsequently had children.

Impotence and family relationships

Impotence obviously exacts a severe toll on personal relationships within the family. The impotence sufferer may feel inner turmoil, and may take his frustration out on his children and his wife, sometimes leading to the severing of family relationships. Reliable statistical data does not exist to permit an analysis of the connection between the high national divorce rate and male sexual dysfunction. But sufficient evidence does exist, in the form of patients' comments, to suggest strongly that there is a connection.

Soap opera mentality provides the popular image of the oversexed, sexually dissatisfied and unsympathetic wife who taunts her husband for his failures and seeks out the services of a readily available stud. This sometimes does occur, as was the case with John and Emily. John, forty-two years old, had experienced coronary bypass surgery. As is often the case in men suffering with arterial disease, the condition extended to the genital area, resulting in his inability to perform sexually. Emily taunted John for his sexual failures and subsequently took a lover. John did not seek help for his sexual dysfunction and eventually died of a heart attack. The emotional strain of impotence and Emily's behavior may have been an important contributory factor in John's death.

Far more typical is the understanding and sympathetic woman, with normal sexual interests, driven to distraction by her partner's anguish and growing panic. In a typical scenario, the female partner may first respond with loving reassurance. As the condition persists, feelings of disappointment and resentment for the denial of pleasure and closeness may develop. The woman may gradually perceive her partner's problem as resulting from her lack of sexuality and physical desirability. Often the woman may suspect that the impotence is a consequence of her partner's active attention to another woman, which leaves him with little physical capacity to spare. Ultimately, the situation may deteriorate to total abstinence, expressions of anger and hostility, and, finally, separation.

Personal health

Male sexual dysfunction frequently goes hand in hand with the deteriorating physical and mental health of both of the involved partners, and even of other members of the family unit. A link between successful sexual performance and low incidence of certain diseases has been noted.

As the physical causes of impotence have become better appreciated, emphasis has shifted to the potentially very serious emotional consequences of impotence. Such consequences may include severe depression, hypochondria, insomnia, alcoholism, drug addiction, and suicide. Self-mutilation by despondent individuals has occurred on occasion.

It is not unusual for afflicted individuals, in desperation, to resort to quack cures, fad diets, gurus, and other assorted charlatans, or to use potentially dangerous chemicals and bizarre mechanical devices. The historical neglect of dysfunction by responsible health care providers is a contributing factor to the widespread prevalence of these fake, and often dangerous, "cures." Zinc supplements, for example, have been heavily touted. A recent advertisement for a zinc supplement promised "bone hard erections." True to form, the advertisement showed the photograph of a smiling, obviously middle-aged man, and an obviously ecstatic young woman. (Zinc deficiency in the United States, incidentally, is not a common problem, nor will zinc supplements restore potency).

At best, a person with a dysfunction may not be physically harmed by these approaches, although valuable time and money is usually lost. At worst, there can be serious consequences. In one recent case, a man had placed a "cock" ring around his penis, in the hope that sufficient rigidity would be provided for intercourse. Use of the device, unfortunately, resulted in severe disfigurement. Numerous cases also exist, in medical literature, of patients who have placed rings and other devices around both the penis and the scrotum, necessitating surgical removal of the rings in hospital emergency rooms.

Job productivity

Patients seeking treatment for sexual dysfunction often complain of difficulties in concentration, frequent mistakes, forgetfulness, impaired judgment, diminished creativity, and loss of drive. In extreme cases, dysfunction can lead to the psychological condition known as abulia, which results in the abnormal lack of ability to act or make decisions. Such conditions can easily result in lowered performance in the workplace, and sometimes even in termination of employment. For the university student suffering from these conditions, academic failure may result.

There is no way to put a price tag on the social cost of diminished worker productivity, but there is little doubt that the cumulative cost to the economy is substantial. Impotence seems to be widely distributed among all occupational groups. It has been suggested, however, that impotence is an especially common affliction among middle-level corporate managers who, as a group, are a major factor in the viability of the economic system. Such individuals are typically highly achievement-oriented and competitive and, as a result, potentially very vulnerable when it comes to sexual failure.

It is possible only to speculate about the broader consequences of sexual dysfunction among individuals in critical occupations, such as the distracted airplane mechanic who forgets to install a vital component, or the key public official suffering from a lack of concentration during a period of international crisis.

Antisocial behavior

There is a story that Adolph Hitler had only one testicle. If this story is true, is it possible that Hitler suffered from a testosterone deficiency contributing to sexual failure? While not much is known about Hitler's sex life, it may be significant that he didn't marry until only a few hours before his death in the Berlin bunker. Some have suggested that Hitler's relationship with his longtime consort, Eva Braun, may have been platonic in nature. In any event, Hitler never had children and apparently had very limited contact with women.

Sexual release is known to have a calming effect on male aggression. It is an open secret that prison officials often encourage situational homosexual behavior. In some more enlightened prisons, conjugal visits are permitted, not only to achieve a more docile convict population, but also as an aid to rehabilitation.

Sexual dysfunction has been suggested as a factor in pederasty, the sexual abuse of children. The pederast, almost always a man, often suffers from performance anxiety. Sex with an adult partner, with normal sexual expectations, could result in great embarrassment were failure to occur. The pederast, therefore, turns to children, where such expectations do not exist, or where the victims may even be too young to understand the nature of the activity.

Obviously, not all men suffering from dysfunction have the evil potential of a Hitler, or commit acts of child abuse. It has been suggested, however, that failure to properly treat afflicted individuals could, on occasion, have very serious social consequences.

Disease symptoms

As impotence may be the consequence of an underlying physical disorder, it follows that the presence of impotence may also be symptomatic of such disorders. For this reason, no thorough physical examination of a patient is complete without systematic inquiry in this area. Unfortunately, this is not often the case. Good medical practice mandates the careful examination of a patient reporting impotence symptoms, especially for possible diabetic and cardiovascular problems. This practice should contribute significantly to the early detection and treatment of such conditions.

Even when impotence can be ultimately linked to psychological factors, prompt investigation of the initial symptoms has been well-justified, since the underlying psychological causes are best identified and treated as early as possible.

HOW MANY MEN ARE IMPOTENT?

If you are being treated for hypertension, there is a possibility that you will become impotent. High blood pressure is a serious medical problem that has received increasing attention in recent years. However, the drug or combination of drugs used to treat hypertension may contribute to impotence. Good medical practice should include a detailed profile of a patient's past sexual performance prior to the start of any treatment. The physician should warn the patient about the side effects of all drugs prescribed, especially those which have been linked to impotence. After treatment is underway, the patient should be closely monitored, and any impotence symptoms must be recorded. Unfortunately, all too often the question of impotence is never discussed unless it is brought up by an aggressive and knowledgeable patient.

So far, there has been very little scientific research into the incidence of male sexual dysfunction, and there is a lack of reliable statistical data on the problem. Dr. William Loomis Furlow, of the Mayo Clinic, estimates the number of American men experiencing chronic impotence (as of 1985), conservatively, at ten million. Furlow's estimate has been calculated from data on the number of men subject to the various health problems that are closely linked to impotence, including diabetes, various vascular diseases, radical pelvic surgery, multiple sclerosis, and spinal cord injuries, plus an allowance for the probable number of men afflicted with impotence of a psychological nature. Many authorities believe that the Furlow estimate is probably too low, and that the actual number could be in the range of twenty to thirty million.

Even if it is assumed that the current number of American impotents is only ten million, the implications are staggering. As of mid-1986, the number of American males eighteen years and older totaled about 84.4 million. Given this figure, roughly 12 percent of all American men are impotent. Stated another way, possibly as many as one out of eight American men is impotent. The next time you are in a large group of men, perhaps on the job or at a sports event, glance around. It may be some small consolation, if you suffer from impotence, to know you are not alone.

Little is known about the prevalence of impotence in the American male population as it relates to such characteristics as ethnic origin, race, and socioeconomic group. Woody Allen, in his hilarious movie, *Sleeper*, depicts a world of the future in which both males and females have lost their sexual powers. Allen's characters had to seek sexual gratification by the use of a mechanical device suggestive of an old-time telephone booth. In Allen's movie, only men of Italian ethnic origin retained their sexual prowess. With all due respect to the Italian stallions among us, this ethnic stereotype has yet to be proven by valid scientific investigation.

Similar stereotypes exist, of course, with respect to American blacks and Hispanics. Black and Hispanic men, nevertheless, frequently turn up at urologists' offices or at impotence support group meetings. It is reasonable to suspect that many of these men bear the additional psychological burden of living up to popular ethnic expectations, as well as the emotional anguish of their underlying condition. Actually, impotence could very well be disproportionately present in both the black and Hispanic communities. In the case of the former, hypertension constitutes a very common problem, and there is also the problem of sickle-cell anemia. In the case of the latter, diabetes is very common.

Very little is known about the incidence of impotence and other male sexual dysfunction problems outside the United States. Third World countries, such as Mexico, Brazil, Nigeria, and India are characterized by relatively young populations and presumably a lower incidence of impotence. The situation in the advanced industrial countries of Western Europe, Japan, and even the Soviet Union probably is similar to that in the United States.

IS IMPOTENCE MORE COMMON TODAY?

A very interesting question is whether impotence and other forms of male sexual dysfunction are becoming more common in the American population. A very popular belief is that the emergence during the late 1960s of the feminist movement and the "new woman" has resulted in an increase in performance anxiety and other psychological factors. There is, however, virtually no tangible scientific evidence to support this view. In addition, there is virtually no reliable information available on the long-term incidence of impotence in the American population.

Several trends, all related to physical rather than psychological causes, however, suggest the strong possibility of a growing impotence problem. One trend is the aging demographic profile of the U.S. population. With the U.S. population growing at a relatively low rate, and the reduced birth rates of recent years, a greater percentage of the male population is now concentrated in the higher age brackets, where impotence is more common. A second factor is the increasing public awareness and concern about high blood pressure, combined with the often indiscriminate prescription of antihypertensive drugs that can lead to impotence. Finally, impotence can be associated with various forms of drug abuse, including alcohol, tobacco, and cocaine, all of which have become increasingly prevalent in our society.

The burden is clearly on the individual sufferer and his partner to obtain proper treatment for male sexual dysfunction. The more knowledgeable the sufferer is, the more aggressive and successful he will be in obtaining proper treatment. Unfortunately, public attitudes and lack of knowledge about the impotence problem are appalling. According to a survey conducted on behalf of the Impotence Information Center and released in 1986, nearly one-half of the general public is reluctant to even discuss the subject, with such reluctance increasing with age. Of those willing to consider the subject, about 45 percent were unable to name a single physical cause of impotence, and 90 percent were totally unaware of the very important diabetes/impotence link. A large segment of the population is unable to properly define impotence, many confuse the concept with infertility, and most are unable to identify the medical specialists who provide treatment.

Impotence sufferers presumably can be expected to be more knowledgeable about the subject. It is, however, not at all uncommon to encounter male patients who have waited many years before seeking treatment. Such individuals often have endured personal tragedy that approaches martyrdom for a condition which, in their ignorance, they tend to blame on themselves. Fortunately, such attitudes may soon be in the past.

Impotence is more than just a sexual problem. Given the importance of male sexuality and the potentially serious consequences of impotence, it is a problem that always should be promptly medically investigated and treated in an appropriate manner. Effective and affordable help is now available for those willing to actively seek assistance.

CHAPTER 2

Impotence
in historical
perspective

D espite the great advances that have been made in recent years in understanding the causes of impotence and other male sexual problems, many incorrect beliefs of the past continue to impact unfavorably on treatment programs. It is helpful for men with impotence problems, and their partners, to become familiar with past beliefs and treatment approaches, in order to be on guard for the possible persistence of antiquated attitudes even among health care professionals.

ANCIENT BELIEFS

Male sexual dysfunction has been a problem since the dawn of history. The ancients typically attributed such problems to the wrath of the gods or the use of witchcraft by enemies. Treatment involved placating the gods with appropriate offerings, or using aphrodisiacs, magic, and the occult.

An Old Testament story (Genesis 20:1-18) has been interpreted as telling of how Abimelech, due to divine intervention, was rendered incapable of successful sexual performance. The minor tribal king's problem had developed following his abduction of Sarah, the wife of the patriarch Abraham. The story has a happy ending, as Abimelech's full powers were restored with the release of Sarah and with the prayers on Abimelech's behalf by, of all people, the wronged husband.

Among the ancient Greeks, it was a common belief that impotence would ultimately be experienced by any man who had been placed on top of a tomb as a child. One possible cure was to take a noxious potion based on the scrapings from the blade of a knife used for gelding rams.

To this day, men still pray to the gods. In Japan, a certain religious shrine is dedicated to male sexual problems. Japanese men, in traditional dress, regularly gather around a large erect wooden penis and seek the help of Shinto deities. Magic potions are still very much in vogue. While on a visit several years ago to Bahia, Brazil, one of the authors was shown, by a high priestess of the African-derived macumba cult, a selection of fearsome-looking preparations suitable for curing impotence. According to the priestess, requests for impotence remedies were about as common as requests for potions to cure intestinal parasites, and were often made by wealthy and highly educated individuals.

ATTITUDES OF NINETEENTH CENTURY MEDICINE

By the nineteenth century, medical science had advanced to the point where a scientific approach to impotence was possible. In fact, as early as the sixteenth century, Varolio, an Italian physician, had observed that the existence of the erection was related to the flow of blood through the penis. Despite great progress in medicine, in general, during the nineteenth century, the treatment of male sexual dysfunction in many ways actually regressed.

The lack of progress can be linked to the highly prudish attitudes toward sex that prevailed during the Victorian era, with such attitudes typified by the use of the word "limbs," instead of "legs," and the strategic placement of fabrics to hide the apparently sexually suggestive legs of tables and chairs. In the supercharged moralistic environment of that period, it was inevitable that the medical establishment would find a connection between impotence and immoral activities, especially masturbation.

A classic statement of the approach of nineteenth century medicine to the impotence problem appears in a fascinating promotional booklet published by a Dr. T. W. Hughes, a licensed physician and surgeon practicing in Atlanta, Georgia, as late as 1926. The seventy-two-page booklet entitled *New Street Guide of Atlanta and Useful Medical Receipts* contains, in addition to a street guide, valuable information on the removal of warts, glowing testimonials to Dr. Hughes, and comments on various medical problems, principally those of a sexual nature. In the exact words of Dr. Hughes, and keeping the original bold type, the passage reads as follows:

> The causes of **Sexual impotency** are as fol-
> lows: **Youthful Follies, Pollutions, (night losses),
> Spermatorrhoea, Prostate Congestion, Gonor-
> rhoea, Stricture, Narrow Meatus** and many
> **Organic Troubles,** such as wasting of the
> **Testicles, Neuralgia of the Testicles, Varicicele,
> Disobedience of Nature's Laws, Sexual Excess or
> Long Abstinence. Sedentary Habits, Worry,
> Anxiety** and **Business Cares,** all tend to produce
> this end, **rendering men powerless and devoid of
> natural function before their time.**

The term "youthful follies," of course, refers to masturbation or "self-abuse." "Pollutions" is a condition characterized by the "too-frequent" occurrence of nocturnal emissions. There is, unfortunately, no explanation provided as to the meaning of the term "disobedience of nature's laws."

The treatment of impotence by the nineteenth century medical establishment was essentially limited to the crusade against masturbation and other moral abominations. Significantly, there is little evidence of any scientific attempt to define the actual physical connection between masturbation and impotence.

Masturbation, incidentally, was blamed for more than just impotence. Among other things, it was the root cause of pollutions. Dr. Hughes would have you believe that boys who masturbate "have a sheepish, hang-dog expression" and "incline to melancholy broodings." Moreover, "their palms are apt to be cold and moist." Adult males who masturbate "are apt to be cowardly, mean-spirited poor specimens of humanity."

It would be a mistake to dismiss these attitudes as merely a nostalgic remembrance of a bygone era. It was only in 1948 that the Boy Scouts of America dropped the famous passage on the evils of masturbation from the pages of their official handbook. Many older men who are today experiencing sexual dysfunction suffer from a residual burden of guilt extending back to exposure to these attitudes in childhood. It is not unreasonable to suspect that many physicians practicing today are still subject to such influences.

TRADITIONAL PSYCHOTHERAPY

The end of the nineteenth century saw the inevitable reaction to prevailing attitudes toward sex, in the work of Sigmund Freud and various associates. Impotence, of course, figures in Freudian thought and is closely related to infantile sexuality, a key element in the Freudian scheme of things. A concise statement of Freud's approach to impotence appeared in an essay "on the Universal Tendency to Debasement in the Sphere of Love," published in 1912. In this essay Freud commented that, following the many forms of anxiety, "psychical" impotence was the most common disorder encountered in psychoanalytical practice. He further noted that the condition could be found in men of a strongly "libidinous" nature, and in men who appear to have no physical conditions that should prevent successful sexual performance.

According to Freud, the explanation for this is the "inhibitory influence of certain psychical complexes." Such complexes are not found in the conscious mind, and hence are not apparent to the individual with the impotence problem. Of the possible complexes, none is more serious than an unresolved incestuous fixation on a mother or perhaps a sister dating back to childhood — in short, the Oedipus complex. Lesser complexes result from traumatic infantile sexual experiences; for example, the shame of a young boy who had been caught in an act of masturbation.

The traditional Freudian approach to the treatment of impotence, in essence is no different than the treatment of any other inhibiting "psychical" (that is, psychological) complex, the now familiar process of psychoanalysis. In psychoanalysis, or the "talking cure," various childhood memories associated with the inhibiting complexes are gradually recalled from memory in extended sessions between the patient and the therapist. Somehow, an awareness of such memories results in the resolution of the complex, along with the eventual disappearance of any related physical and emotional problems.

In a relatively short period of time, traditional Freudian psychoanalysis would fragment into a spectrum of contentious and often pseudoscientific cults. Wide variations in treatment approaches also emerged, ranging from group therapy to hypnotherapy to primal scream therapy. It was increasingly acknowledged, by all but the strictest followers of classic Freudian dogma, that factors, other than just those associated with incest and infant sexuality, might result in impotence and other problems. At the same time, the idea that impotence was essentially "all in the head" became a fixed belief, not only among psychotherapists, but also throughout the general medical establishment. Little scientific interest was shown in the possible biological mechanisms by which problems "in the head" somehow result in a lack of physical performance in the penis.

By 1927, Wilhelm Stekel, a prominent European neuropsychiatrist and psychotherapist, was able to claim that practically all cases of impotence were linked to psychic inhibitions that could be treated with psychotherapy. Moreover, Stekel went on to theorize that underlying the psychic inhibitions resulting in impotence are various cultural forces, such as religion, the family, and the political and economic system. Such views, unfortunately, are at odds with the obvious existence of many sexually capable men in the most restrictive segments of modern society, and the frequent discovery of impotent men in primitive societies where there are no restrictive institutions.

Despite increasing evidence of the shortcomings of "all- in-the-head" theories, David Reuben, M.D., in 1969, could still categorically state in the highly successful best seller *Everything You Always Wanted to Know About Sex but Were Afraid to Ask*: "There is convincing evidence that the source of male potency is in the brain."[1] Reuben went on to acknowledge, however, that about 5 percent of all impotence has a physical basis. As to a possible cure for an impotence problem, Reuben suggested only psychiatry and hypnosis.

Despite the major advances in understanding and treating impotence in the past several decades, *The Complete Manual of Fitness and Well-Being*, published in 1984, could advise, "Impotence is mainly a psychological phenomenon caused by external stresses." As to treatment, the book assured readers that, "Once these have been removed, potency usually returns."[2]

---

[1] David R. Reuben, *Everything You Always Wanted to Know About Sex but Were Afraid to Ask* (New York: McKay Co., 1969), pp. 98-99.

[2] Robert Arnot, M.D., Special Advisor, *The Complete Manual of Fitness and Well-Being* (New York: Viking, 1984), p. 165.

THE ERA OF SEX THERAPY

Until very recently, the subject of human sexuality received short shrift at most medical schools and in the general scientific community. The problem of impotence in particular was not investigated from a medical viewpoint. Those researchers who did study sexuality were wedded to traditional psychoanalytical approaches, which prevented them from conducting systematic scientific investigations.

In 1966, the results of over ten years of research by William H. Masters, M.D., Virginia E. Johnson, and others at the Reproductive Biology Research Foundation, St. Louis, Missouri, appeared in the book *Human Sexual Response*.[3] Despite the highly technical nature of the findings, the book caused an immediate sensation. Unfortunately, an undeniable factor in the book's success was the public's titillation with the experimental methods employed in the research project, such as direct observation of the actual sexual performance of male and female volunteers, and the use of cameras, cardiographs, blood monitors, and other laboratory devices. In 1970, Masters and Johnson followed up with a second book, *Human Sexual Inadequacy*, which dealt specifically with problems of sexual dysfunction in both males and females. This time the public was treated to reports of the use of sexual "surrogates" in the experimental program.[4]

The Masters and Johnson studies must be regarded as a major milestone in the understanding of how erotic stimulation impacts on the human body anatomically and physiologically. They have also provided some useful information on sexual dysfunction. On the other hand, the studies have tended to perpetuate the traditional belief that impotence is essentially a psychological problem. It is important to observe, however, that the original Masters

---

[3] William H. Masters and Virginia E. Johnson, *Human Sexual Response* (Boston: Little, Brown & Co., 1966).

[4] William H. Masters and Virginia E. Johnson, *Human Sexual Inadequacy* (Boston: Little, Brown & Co., 1970).

and Johnson studies concede the possibility of physical causes of impotence, at least in some cases.

A key belief in the Masters and Johnson system is that a variety of psychological stress factors result in impotence. "Performance anxiety," or the excessive fear of the consequences of unsuccessful sexual performance, is singled out as especially important. Performance anxiety, moreover, is believed to be self-reinforcing, with episodes of failure resulting in cycles of heightened anxiety and repeated failure.

The Masters and Johnson studies, however, provided little insight into the actual mechanism at work within the human body by which fears and anxieties centered in the brain result in the loss of erection. Some observers have suggested that performance anxiety could trigger surges of the chemical epinephrine, better known as adrenalin, into the bloodstream. This, in turn, could result in a diminished flow of blood to the penis and loss of erection.

Treatment methods based on the Masters and Johnson theories of sexual dysfunction typically involve an active approach, which ranges from masturbation exercises to participation by the sexual partners in various exercises including touching, fondling, and so forth. This approach has been labeled "sensate focus" therapy. The emphasis in sensate focus therapy is on direct behavioral reconditioning in the present, rather than the intensive probing of the past. Through behavioral modification, it is hoped that cures can be achieved in a matter of months, rather than the many years characteristic of traditional psychotherapy.

One major consequence of the Masters and Johnson studies has been the emergence of "sex therapy" as a generally recognized field of professional specialization. The practitioners, or "sex therapists," are a diverse group, including individuals with traditional medical training, psychologists, and others with varying backgrounds in personal and family counseling. In general, most sex therapists are strongly influenced by the Masters and Johnson explanations of sexual dysfunction, and their suggested treatment approaches. There is, however, a significant and growing number of sex therapists who recognize the importance of physical factors in impotence.

TREATMENT WITH DRUGS AND SURGERY

The restraints of traditional psychotherapy, combined with contemporary sex therapy approaches and a more hospitable environment for human sexuality research, have served to stimulate medical inquiry into treatments involving surgery and drugs. Research in the field, however, dates back a long way.

Research on penile injections can be traced back to 1668 when Regneri de Graaf, by injecting fluid through a syringe, performed a "miracle," raising an erection in the penis of a cadaver. Hormonal treatment dates to at least 1889 when Frenchman Brown-Sequard injected himself with an extract from the testicles of dogs and noted that he was well pleased with the results. Public interest in hormonal therapy was aroused when, in 1918, another researcher working in France, Serge Voronoff, reported that youth could be prolonged by the grafting of cells from monkey testicles into men. For many years, the public was regularly treated to sensationalized stories of the possibility of renewed youth from the use of "monkey glands." It is difficult to trace the use of surgery to correct impotence associated with vascular problems or physical injuries, but by the mid-1930s several successful operations of this nature were reported.

Penile implants date at least to the 1930s. In 1936, N.A. Bogoras, a Russian, used a section of cartilage from a patient's ribs to reconstruct a penis that had been accidentally amputated. The reconstructed penis was reported to have adequate rigidity for intercourse. Implants based on synthetic materials can be traced to the early 1950s. Research on penile implants accelerated in the 1960s. By the 1970s, standard devices for penile implantation were available on a commercial basis.

Recent advances in the use of drugs and surgery have resulted in practical solutions to the problem of physical impotence. Apart from the selected use of the penile implant, and the penile injection of a drug known as papaverine, there are still no surgical or pharmaceutical solutions to the problem of true psychological impotence. Research now underway could offer long-range alternatives to extended psychotherapy or sex therapy. Assuming the validity of the theory that psychological impotence results from excessive fear-induced adrenalin production, the use of various substances to block adrenalin output by the adrenal gland might serve as a solution. Such substances are known to exist, although there is concern as to side effects. It is also potentially dangerous to completely block the adrenalin supply, considering adrenalin's importance in the body's normal response to emergency situations.

After thousands of years, impotence is finally coming out of the closet. The focus has finally shifted from unsupported psychological speculation, blaming the victim for supposed youthful follies, to experimental research and the application of the scientific method. As a result, more has been learned in the past several decades about the causes and effective treatment of impotence than was learned in the past several centuries.

CHAPTER 3

Understanding the male sexual mechanism

U nderstanding the causes of impotence and other male sexual problems requires some basic knowledge of the design of the male sexual mechanism and the physical events that should normally take place during sexual intercourse.

Several diagrams in this chapter help explain the mechanical aspects of male sexual behavior. The first diagram, Figure 3-1, shows the various components of the male urinary-genital system, and how they are interconnected. Figure 3-2 shows, in highly simplified form, the all-important vascular or blood supply connections to the interior of the penis. The third diagram, Figure 3-3, reveals the internal structure of the penis, and includes the key elements within the penis that make erection possible.

THE MALE URINARY-GENITAL SYSTEM

As its name implies, the male urinary-genital system serves more than one purpose. One of its purposes is to

24

provide the means for the necessary and continuing elimination of liquid wastes from the body in the form of urine. A second purpose is to provide the means for the male contribution to the process of human reproduction. The urinary-genital system also includes facilities that manufacture the vital chemical substances that are critical to growth (especially during puberty), and that contribute to general good health and vigor.

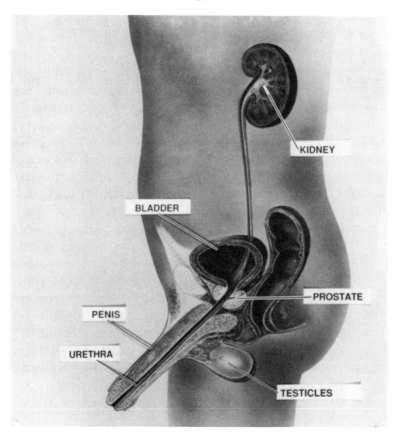

Figure 3-1
Components of the Male Urinary-Genital System
Courtesy of Bard Urological Division, C.R. Bard, Inc.
Illustration by Anthony E. Foote

A discussion of the individual components of the male urinary-genital system and their respective functions follows. Also see Figure 3-1 for an illustration of the various components of the male urinary-genital system.

The penis

The penis is used both for the elimination of urine and for reproduction. Over the course of a lifetime, the penis is obviously used most of the time for urine elimination. In urination, the penis is an important component of the pathway for the flow of urine from the bladder to the outside of the body. In reproduction, the penis serves as the pathway for sperm and spermatic fluid to the outside of the body. It also serves, when in the erect state, as the means for the deposition of sperm at a point within the female body where the chances for successful impregnation are the greatest. Finally, the penis is the site where most of the pleasurable physical sensations associated with intercourse and orgasm are concentrated. Such pleasurable sensations, in both men and women, apparently serve to encourage frequent intercourse and hence insure the propagation of the human species.

Many men are unnecessarily concerned about penis size. In one scientific investigation, the average nonerect penis length, in a group of fifty men aged eighteen to fifty-three, was found to be only 9.4 centimeters (about 3.5 inches). At the same time, the average penis diameter for the group was only 2.9 centimeters (slightly over an inch). There is no evidence that men with smaller penis dimensions are at any tangible disadvantage with respect to sexual performance.

The testicles

The testicles serve as the site for the production of sperm and male sexual hormones, especially testosterone. An adequate supply of healthy sperm is a critical element in the reproductive process. Sperm, however, is not a factor in the impotence problem. Men with low sperm counts and men who have chosen to have vasectomies are perfectly capable of highly successful sexual intercourse, that is, they are capable of having erections and of successful vaginal penetration. Contrary to popular folklore, the existence of a large family by no means implies extraordinary virility.

Testosterone is a steroid substance that plays a very important role in the processes that take place in young men during puberty. An inadequate testosterone supply at this stage of life can result in the failure to develop such normal masculine characteristics as facial and body hair and the typically deep male speaking voice. In older men, an inadequate supply of testosterone is often associated with a loss of libido or sexual desire, and sometimes with the failure to obtain and maintain an erection. Such men may also experience muscular weakness and a general loss of vigor.

The location of the testicles outside the body, in the pouch known as the scrotum, reflects the fact that ideal conditions for sperm production are at temperatures below the normal body temperature of 98.6° F. Cold temperatures do not inhibit sperm production. Remember that collected sperm is often stored frozen and later thawed for artificial insemination. The location of the testicles outside the body cavity does, however, make them more prone to physical injury.

Testicles are formed within the body of the fetus, and sometimes one or even both testicles have not descended into the scrotum at the time of birth. This condition can usually be easily corrected. Incidentally, one testicle normally hangs slightly lower than the other. This configuration reflects a certain lack of symmetry in the internal structure of the human body.

The prostate and seminal vesicles

The prostate is a single gland, unique to men, which is located in a highly confined position under the bladder and in close proximity to the urethra. The prostate serves as the source of about one-half of the whitish fluid known as semen, which carries the sperm. Two glands, known as the seminal vesicles, account for the additional fluid that makes up the semen. These glands are located behind the prostate.

The prostate is a frequent source of a variety of problems men may face as they age. Physicians examine the prostate by means of a finger inserted through the rectum.

The vas deferens

Two lengthy tubular structures known as the vas deferens are connected to each testicle and serve as parallel pipelines for the delivery of sperm out of the testicles. The fluid flowing from each vas deferens flows into two intersections analogous to the "T-joints" in plumbing systems. At the T-joints, the fluid originating in the testicles joins and mixes with fluid flowing from each seminal vesicle. The joint stream, plus additional fluid originating in the prostate, ultimately flows through a channel to the urethra.

The surgical severing and tying of each vas deferens constitutes the now-common operative procedure known as a vasectomy. With each vas deferens severed, sperm cannot travel out of the testicles and the patient, by choice, is rendered infertile. Following a vasectomy, the sperm that continues to be generated in the testicles has no place to go and is harmlessly absorbed in the body. Normal ejaculation of semen, and orgasm, however, continue as before the operation.

A vasectomy in no way affects the production of testosterone or its distribution throughout the body, because the normal route for the movement of testosterone out of the testicles is through the blood system. In short, it is impossible for a vasectomy to physically affect sexual performance.

The bladder

Because the kidney generates urine on a continuous basis and humans urinate only intermittently, a facility is required for temporary urine storage. This is provided by the sac-like structure known as the bladder.

In urination, urine leaving the bladder passes through another plumbing-type T-joint and subsequently leaves the body via the penis. During periods of sexual activity, ejaculatory fluid also flows through this T-joint. The passage of urine through the "T," however, is controlled by the sphincter muscle, which acts as a valve to prevent the passage of urine during sexual intercourse as well as the backup of ejaculatory fluid into the bladder.

The urethra

The urethra serves as a joint pipeline for the movement of both urine and ejaculatory fluid through the penis to the tip of the penis, where it can exit the body. Most of the length of the urethra is contained within the penis, although it commences well within the pelvic cavity.

During urination, urine normally flows rapidly through the urethra in a strong continuous stream until the bladder is emptied. Various problems, such as an enlarged prostate, can impede flow. During periods of sexual activity, the urethra serves as a temporary holding space where ejaculatory fluid can collect prior to expulsion during ejaculation.

THE BLOOD SUPPLY
TO THE PENIS

The importance of the blood supply to the penis cannot be overemphasized. Figure 3-2 shows a simplified diagram of the blood supply to the penis. The blood supply to any part of the body, of course, is critical, in view of the role of the blood in the supply of nutrients and oxygen to the tissues, the removal of waste products, and the transport of immunological agents, hormones, and other essential chemical entities. In the case of the penis, the blood supply serves a unique function. As will be discussed in detail, blood acts as a hydraulic fluid which makes penile erection possible.

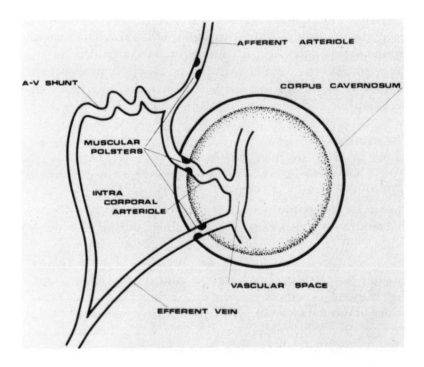

Figure 3-2
Simplified Diagram of the Blood Supply to the Penis

Blood is pumped to the penis by the heart through the same arterial system that supplies the legs and other locations in the lower body. As the blood moves downstream, it branches out into the large penile artery. This artery then splits within the penis into three major paired arterial systems: the deep artery system, the dorsal artery system, and the bulbosa artery system. Each of these systems in turn branches into innumerable channels, which supply various portions of the penis.

The dorsal arteries and associated dorsal veins are familiar to most men, since they can be faintly seen under the skin of the penis. The deep arteries, however, are the most important in erection, because they supply blood to the tissues known as the corpus cavernosum, the site of the erectile process.

While arteries carry blood upstream into the penis, veins carry blood downstream from the penis through what is known as the venous blood system, and back to the heart. The extensive network of veins within the corpus cavernosum is also believed to play a key role in the erection process.

THE NERVE SUPPLY
TO THE PENIS

Autonomic (unconscious) and somatic (conscious) nerve circuits interconnect the penis with nerve centers in the brain and key nerve bundles in the spinal column. Electrical impulses provide the means for the transmission of information through the nerve circuits. It is interesting to note in this connection that ejaculation has been experimentally achieved by stimulation from an external electrical source.

The autonomic and somatic nervous systems both play a role in the erection process. The autonomic system is divided into two subsystems, the parasympathetic and the sympathetic. The former subsystem is involved in the unconscious processes associated with initiating erection. The somatic nervous system serves as the electrical pathway for the transmission of conscious erotic images, including the pleasurable sensations associated with sexual activities.

THE MECHANICS OF ERECTION

Erection and ejaculation should not be confused. Erection is necessary in order to provide the penis with sufficient rigidity to permit the penetration of the female vagina. Ejaculation, however, can be achieved by masturbation in the absence of an erection, although this implies a loss of much of the pleasure associated with sexual relations, and presents obvious problems with respect to having children.

In humans, erection is achieved by a hydraulic mechanism. Hydraulic systems are based on the difficulty of compressing a liquid. As a result, when a force is applied to a liquid confined within a limited area, a buildup of pressure occurs and the liquid will press against its physical boundaries.

The brake systems found in modern automobiles are hydraulic in nature. When the driver presses the brake pedal, the considerable pressure buildup activates the braking process. Hydraulic brake systems normally work very well, and for this reason were adopted many years ago for use in automobiles. As every driver knows, hydraulic brakes sometimes fail, particularly when leaks occur in the vicinity of the seals. With the penis, leakage of hydraulic fluid, in this case blood, is one of the possible causes of loss of an erection.

Incidentally, some types of whales do not employ the hydraulic approach for the formidable task of coitus on the high seas. Instead, such whales are equipped with a penile bone. Many men are now employing something very similar, in the form of a penile implant.

In order to understand how hydraulic forces make an erection possible, it is useful to examine Figure 3-3, the diagram showing the internal structure of the penis. As can be seen from the diagram, "corpus cavernosa" tissue, shaped into two long cylinders, parallels the shaft of the penis over most of its length. When conditions call for an erection, these tissue structures absorb large quantities of

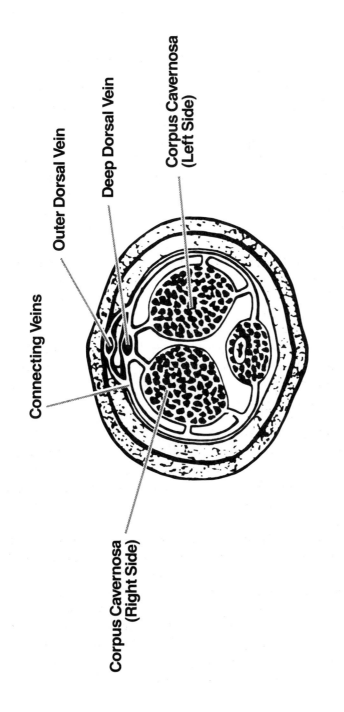

Figure 3-3
Internal Structure of the Penis
Courtesy of Bard Urological Division, C.R. Bard, Inc.
Illustration by Anthony E. Foote

the hydraulic fluid (blood), resulting in the expansion of penis length, diameter, and needed rigidity.

Within the corpus cavernosum are thousands of expandable sac-like structures, known as sinuses, each capable of storing very large quantities of blood. Exactly how these structures fill with blood during an erection is still subject to some uncertainty, although research may soon provide a full explanation. From the standpoint of hydraulics, filling the sinuses with blood logically involves the continuous pumping of upstream or arterial blood into the sinus cavities, and some form of valving action to restrict the downstream movement of blood from the cavities into the veins of the venous blood system. One suggested explanation is that as the sinuses fill with blood, they press against the veins and restrict all or most of the downstream flow. This does not account, however, for how the buildup of blood in the sinuses occurs in the first place.

One possible way to increase the flow of blood into the sinuses would be to substantially increase the pumping rate of the heart. The variations in heartbeat that occur during periods of sexual activity are not sufficient in themselves to account for the buildup of blood in the sinuses. A more likely explanation is that the flow of blood into the sinuses is enhanced due to the action of muscle tissues located within the corpus cavernosum. There is also evidence of a major increase in the internal blood pressure of the corpus cavernosum, to well above normal body readings, during erection.

What appears most likely is that the erection gets underway when the involved muscles first vigorously contract. This, in turn, serves to dilate (increase the diameter) of the arteries entering the corpus cavernosum, resulting in increased blood flow. Then, as the erection process gains momentum, the valving action in the exiting veins may come into play. It is also reasonable to conclude that feedback relationships probably exist between the indicated upstream and downstream mechanisms.

Of course, an erection will not occur unless appropriate messages are sent to the nerve centers in the penis that directly control the muscles of the corpus cavernosum. The erection is essentially a reflex action that cannot be consciously willed. Sometimes an erection is triggered by psychological factors when the center in the brain associated with the functions of the somatic nervous system is activated by intimate contact with a sexual partner or by merely viewing or even imagining erotic images. An erection may also be triggered, via the parasympathetic nervous system, when nerve centers located in the spinal cord are stimulated by the physical stroking of the penis. Typically, both processes take place simultaneously. It is also typical, as men age, for the erection to become more dependent upon direct physical stimulation of the penis, a factor that should be recognized during sexual relations.

Erections are, of course, expected to take place during periods of sexual activities with a partner, or during masturbation. In healthy men, erections also normally occur about three to six times per night, while asleep and during dream periods. Such nocturnal erections may last for up to thirty minutes, and are often observed by men when awakening. Studies have shown that nocturnal erections can often occur during dreams that have no erotic content. This seems to indicate that nocturnal erections are largely controlled by the autonomic nervous system.

The reasons for nocturnal erections are not fully known, but such erections may represent the way the body checks on whether the erectile mechanism is working properly, in much the same manner that aerospace engineers repeatedly check key mechanical systems prior to launching a complicated space vehicle.

THE MECHANICS OF EJACULATION

Ejaculation occurs as a result of vigorous contractions of muscles in the vicinity of the urethra and in the pelvic area. The pumping action provided by the contractions is similar to what occurs at the beach when you quickly squeeze the surface of the water with a cupped hand and observe the resulting upright spurt.

The contractions causing the expulsion of seminal fluid are reflexes that are neurological in nature and normally extend to the area of the anus. The completed interrelation of nerve connections in this general area serves as the basis for several tests discussed in Chapter 5, which may be easily performed in the privacy of the home.

Prior to the moment of ejaculation, a quantity of semen collects in the urethra. The channel connecting the urethra to the bladder is normally closed by the sphincter muscle, while the pathways upstream through the vas deferens are too small to permit reverse fluid flow. Under these circumstances, the muscular contractions can only result in the movement of fluid downstream, through the urethra and out the tip of the penis.

The pleasurable sensations that take place during ejaculation are not dependent upon the presence of the semen. Surgical removal of the prostate results in the absence of the ejaculatory fluid. It is, nevertheless, still possible to experience the physical sensations of ejaculation, provided there has been minimal damage to critical nerve connections.

The pleasurable sensations that occur at the moment of ejaculation are, of course, those associated with male orgasm. In the Masters and Johnson studies of the 1960s, a male sexual response cycle was defined, in which the events that take place during sexual activities are divided into successive "excitement," "plateau," "orgasm," and "resolution" stages. In orgasm, two substages have been identified: a period of ejaculatory inevitability and a period of actual ejaculation. The short period of ejaculatory inevitability is believed to take place at the time when substantial quantities of semen collect in the urethra. The awareness that ejaculation is imminent and irreversible is a very familiar feeling to most men.

During the resolution stage that follows ejaculation, the erection is normally quickly lost. In the shutdown process, nerve impulses direct the relaxation of the muscles of the corpus cavernosum. This results, in turn, in the decreased flow of upstream arterial blood, the collapse of the sinus cavities, and the rapid downstream flow of the blood that had been temporarily stored within the penis.

THINGS THAT CAN GO WRONG

The male urinary-genital system normally works remarkably well, considering its overall complexity and restricted geometry. However, one inherent design flaw is the combination of the urinary and genital functions. As any engineer can attest, the tying together of functional systems in any complicated device, such as an automobile, means that a failure in one system will, more than likely, result in trouble in all the other interrelated systems, and possibly total incapacitation. The female body, incidentally, is more logically designed, in that there is a complete separation of the equipment used for urination and that used for reproduction.

The tight geometry of the male urinary-genital system results in problems similar to those faced by the automobile mechanic working under the crowded hood of a modern motor vehicle. In this respect, men do have an advantage over women — in the female body there is even less space to work in when something goes wrong.

Impotence has always been the most common problem of the male urinary-genital system with respect to successful sexual performance. The causes of impotence are discussed in the next chapter. There are other problems that men experience, such as premature ejaculation, that can often be just as troubling. These problems, which are discussed in Chapter 5, may have a serious impact on health and well-being. Examples include infections of the prostate and urethra; tumors of the prostate, testicles, and bladder;

kidney stones; the general problem of male infertility. While a general discussion of these problems is beyond the scope of this book, some of these problems can contribute to dysfunction and are relevant in this sense.

Any patient diagnosed as having one of the above problems would be well-advised to bear in mind the possibility of a connection between his medical condition and impotence, and certainly should discuss this with his doctor if he has any of the symptoms of impotence.

CHAPTER 4

What causes impotence

Given the way erection takes place, it is logical to conclude that impotence is essentially a problem caused by one or more negative factors impacting in some way on the blood supply or nerve connections to the penis. In some cases, a single factor affecting either the blood supply or the nerve connections may underlie the problem. Other cases may be more complicated, with multiple factors at work. The possibility of impotence of a psychological nature is by no means precluded. When psychological factors are at work, they can be manifested only via chemical agents transported through the bloodstream or electrical impulses transmitted via the nervous system.

The problems that are known to cause impotence under some circumstances may be logically grouped as follows:

- Problems that mainly affect the blood supply
- Problems that mainly affect the nervous system
- Other problems that significantly affect both systems, or those in which the mechanism is currently not fully understood

BLOOD SUPPLY PROBLEMS

Blood supply, or "vasculogenic," problems that may adversely affect erection occur on either the upstream (arterial) side of the penis, or on the downsteam (venous) side. On the upstream side, it is reasonable to suspect anything that diminishes the flow of arterial blood to the penis as a possible cause of impotence. These include the following:

- Constriction of arteries
- Blockage of arteries
- Thickening of the blood

On the downstream side, abnormal leakage of blood out of the sinus cavities can result in impotence. A number of factors may account for such leakage.

Constriction of arteries

In the typical male, the average inside diameter of each of the deep penile arteries that supply blood to the corpus cavernosum is in the 1.5 to 3.0 millimeter (about 0.06 to 0.12 inch) range. At the lower end of the range, the diameter is smaller than the head of a pin. Because these tight dimensions provide very little excess flow capacity, any further reduction in size is capable of causing problems. Some men are also just born with very narrow arteries, and unfortunately may have a potential problem built into their systems.

Arteriosclerosis, a leading cause of death in older men and women, is also a major factor underlying male impotence. In the very common form of arteriosclerosis popularly known as hardening of the arteries, the interior arterial walls throughout the body gradually become lined with deposits of fatty substances over a period of time. This buildup of deposits results in both a constriction of the lumen, or inside arterial channel, and a decrease in arterial elasticity. Under these circumstances, there is a reduction in the normal flow of blood through the flaccid or nonerect penis. Even worse, the penile arteries will not sufficiently dilate to permit increased blood flow when the signal arrives through the nervous system calling for an erection.

The use of tobacco products, especially cigarettes, has been clearly linked to both impotence and the increased statistical risk of heart disease. Substances in tobacco smoke have been found to cause significant blood vessel constriction. On occasion, some impotence patients have even experienced greatly improved erectile function following the cessation of smoking. The male smoker therefore faces the increased long-range risk of becoming impotent, due to the consequences of heart disease, and a more immediate risk from the direct effects of tobacco.

Radiation therapy in the vicinity of the penis can result in impotence. Radiation therapy is often called for in cases of cancer of the prostate or bladder. About 40 percent of the men who are treated with radiation therapy for a prostate carcinoma report some degree of erectile difficulty. Scarring of tissue in all forms of radiation therapy is very common. When the blood vessels of the penis are scarred, they greatly lose the elasticity needed for proper penile blood flow during erections.

Blockage of arteries

Impotence can result from any significant blockage at a critical point in the major arteries serving the penis. Blockages can result from operative procedures, physical injury, and the aging process. Whenever surgery is performed on the major blood vessels of the body, there is a danger of a small fatty deposit, known as an embolus, breaking loose, flowing downstream, and lodging at some point, thus creating a blockage.

Blockages can result from some physical injuries to the pelvic region that result in obstruction of one or more of the major arteries. With age, blockages can occur in the major blood vessels leading to the legs. Such blockages can result in difficulty walking. Since the arteries to the penis split off from the arteries leading to the legs, it is very common for men experiencing such blockages to simultaneously experience problems with erections.

Thickening of the blood

Decreased flow of blood to the penis may occur in conditions that result in a thickening or loss of fluidity of the blood. Blood can take on a sludge-like character in individuals suffering from sickle-cell anemia, a genetic disease largely experienced by persons of African and Mediterranean ancestry. Chemotherapy, used in the treatment of certain kinds of cancer, can also result in a similar effect on blood.

Abnormal leakage of blood

Men subject to leakage of venous blood from the sinus cavities often experience semirigid erections and erections that are quickly lost. A condition known as an arterial venous malformation, in which there is a defective connection between the arteries and the veins, may be at the root of the problem. Defective valving action on the venous side, or inadequate filling of the sinus cavities, can also be a factor.

PROBLEMS IN THE
NERVOUS SYSTEM

The following problems primarily affecting the nervous system have been identified as possible causes of impotence:

- Alcohol abuse
- Illegal substance abuse
- Use of certain prescription and nonprescription drugs
- Surgery and physical injury
- Neurological disorders
- Psychological factors

Chapter 5 describes some simple tests that you can perform yourself to determine whether you have suffered nerve damage.

Alcohol abuse

The abuse of alcohol can play a very significant role in impotence. Moderate alcohol consumption has been said to have an aphrodisiac effect. In moderation, the effect can be an increase in libido and the reduction of social and sexual inhibitions. With heavier drinking, the central nervous system is subject to depression, and the drinker typically experiences some loss of control over mental and physical faculties. Even younger men in excellent health and with no history of sexual dysfunction can experience episodes of temporary impotence when drunk. Such situations only reconfirm the sad truth of Shakespeare's words, that alcohol "provokes the desire, but takes away the performance" (*Macbeth*, Act II, Scene 3).

Moderate social drinking does not seem to represent a major contributory factor to chronic persistent impotence. At some point, however, a significant portion of the population crosses the line between moderate social drinking and the alcohol dependency syndrome better known as alcoholism. The usual symptoms of alcoholism are early morning drinking, consistent heavy daily intake, and withdrawal symptoms during periods of abstinence. Perhaps as many as 5 percent of the U.S. male population typically become alcoholics, probably as a consequence of their inherent metabolic profiles.

Alcoholism in both men and women frequently results in serious impairment of the peripheral nervous system. Damage is cumulative, and in males extends to the nerves controlling the bulbocavernosus reflex in the penis. The result can be irreversible damage that will continue into the future despite regained sobriety.

Alcoholism also takes its toll as a result of its typical effect on the body's hormonal balances. High estrogen and low testosterone levels are often detected in male alcoholics. The liver, an organ often seriously damaged by alcohol abuse, can be an important factor in this occurrence. As the normal function of the liver is impaired, the level of the female hormone, estrogen, rises in the bloodstream. At the same time, testosterone levels drop, due to the increased breakdown of the male hormone by the liver. Alcohol also inhibits the production of testosterone in the testicles. As a result, testosterone levels may be reduced even in the absence of severe liver damage.

The hormonal abnormalities that are often seen in male alcoholics can clearly have an impact on sexual characteristics and function. For example, noticeable breast and nipple enlargement often takes place in chronic alcohol abusers.

The impotent alcoholic's difficulties are often compounded by heavy smoking, use of various illegal substances, poor diet, and overeating. The combination frequently has synergistic consequences that work together to exacerbate the problem. Overeating, leading to obesity, is often associated with heart disease and high blood pressure. The medications used to treat these problems often result in impotence. Finally, the usual pattern of vitamin deficiency and emotional stress in male alcoholics may also add to the impotence problem.

This combination of problems that often exists for the male alcoholic is illustrated by the profile of George, age sixty, who was treated for impotence. George, a construction worker, reported that it is very common for workers in the building trades to drink heavily on the job. In fact, many employers routinely provide large quantities of beer, in the belief that this stimulates production. George has had previous surgery for prostate cancer and had been taking prescription drugs linked to impotence to treat high blood pressure and ulcers. A penile implant proved the only solution for his impotence.

Illegal substance abuse

All of the common mind-altering substances usually bought and consumed on an illegal basis are suspect when it comes to impotence. The level of use at which problems will develop with these substances is even less clear than with alcohol, given the obvious impediments to scientific research in this area.

Marijuana (cannabis), the most widely used illegal substance, is relatively benign with respect to impotence and, in general, appears to present less of a problem than alcohol. Use of marijuana and associated substances, such as hashish, does lower testosterone levels and can inhibit normal erections. Fortunately, the effect on testosterone is usually short term and reversible. It is worth noting, however, that there are reports in the medical literature linking impotence to long-term marijuana use.

The use of cocaine (known in concentrated form as crack) may lead to serious impotence problems. Male cocaine users sometimes report increased libido the first few times the drug is consumed. Long-term habitual users, however, very often report partial or complete loss of erection. The drug is known to have an adverse effect on the central and peripheral nervous systems. Amphetamines, such as speed have similar effects on the central and peripheral nervous systems, and are also implicated in impotence.

Opium derivatives, such as heroin, are believed to act as aphrodisiacs in very small doses. Consumption of larger quantities and habitual use can result in decreased libido and nervous system damage contributing to impotence. Similar problems may result from methadone, a synthetic heroin substitute that is often legally provided to narcotics abusers in treatment programs.

Use of certain prescription and nonprescription drugs

Impotence is a possible side effect of a broad spectrum of drugs commonly used in the treatment of various medical problems. Most of the time such drugs are available only on a prescription basis; however, problems can exist with some drugs sold without prescription on an over-the-counter basis. A listing of products to be aware of is provided beginning on page 47.

Problems are most common in the case of cardiovascular preparations, which include drugs used in the treatment of high blood pressure and various heart and vascular system problems. Frequently prescribed brand-name drugs in which impotence problems have been encountered include Aldomet, Serpasil, Inderal, and Lopressor. Exactly how the various cardiovascular preparations act to cause impotence is still not fully understood, and the exact mechanism may also vary from drug to drug. It has been suggested that many drugs of this type inhibit the normal function of the neurotransmitters that control the dilation of the critical blood vessels of the corpus cavernosum.

Many drugs used for the control of emotional states have been linked to impotence. These include tranquilizers and antianxiety preparation ("downers"), and antidepressants ("uppers"). In the former category are such brand-name products as Valium, Librium, Equanil, and Thorazine. The latter category includes such brand-name drugs as Elavil and Tofranil. It is worth noting that depression is a frequent side effect of drugs used to treat high blood pressure. Such circumstances may present a patient with a double impotence risk.

A partial list of the types of drugs that have also been linked to impotence includes barbiturates, sedatives, sleeping pills, and antihistamines. These drugs are believed to alter, in some manner, the proper functioning of the central nervous system. The widely prescribed brand-name drug, Tagamet, used in the treatment of ulcers, has been linked to impotence. Other side effects of the drug may include decreased libido and lethargy. The effects of the drug are a result of the increased levels of the hormone, prolactin.

Estrogen therapy is frequently employed in the treatment of cancer of the prostate. Typical effects of use of the female hormone are reduced libido and impotence. Estrogen has often been employed in quack cures for male baldness. Most of these cures have fortunately involved the use of the hormone in salves and lotions applied to the skin on a topical basis. As such, they have probably not contributed to impotence. They have also not contributed to the desired growth of hair.

FREQUENTLY USED DRUGS LINKED TO IMPOTENCE[1]

Cardiovascular Drugs (for High Blood Pressure, Heart Disease, Cholesterol Control, and Related Problems)

Generic (Technical) Name	*Brand Name(s)*
Chlorthalidone	Combipres, Demi-Regroton, Hygroton
Chlorothiazide	Diuril
Clofibrate	Altromid-S
Clonidine hydrochloride	Catapres, Combipres

Cardiovascular Drugs (for High Blood Pressure, Heart Disease, Cholesterol Control, and Related Problems)
(Continued)

Generic (Technical) Name	*Brand Name(s)*
Digitalis	Crystodigen
Digoxin	Lanoxicaps, Lanoxin
Disopyramide phosphate	Norpace
Guanethidine sulfate	Esimil, Ismelin
Hydrochlorothiazide	Aldactazide, Aldoril, Apesazide, Dyazide, Esidrix, Esimil, HydroDiuril, Hydropres, Inderide, Moduretic Tablets, Ser-Ap-Es
Metoprolol	Lopressor
Methylodopa	Aldoclor, Aldomet, Aldoril
Pargyline hydrochloride	Eutonyl, Eutron
Phenoxybenzamine hydrochloride	Dibenzyline
Phentolamine	Regitine
Propranolol	Inderal, Inderide
Rauwolfia serpentina	Harmonyl, Raudixin, Rauzide Tablets
Reserpine	Demi-Regroton, Diupres, Hydropres, Metatesin, Regroton, Salutesin, Sandril, Ser-Ap-Es, Serpasil
Spironolactone	Aldactazine, Aldactone

Drugs for Controlling the Emotions (Tranquilizers, Antidepressants, Antianxiety Agents)

Generic (Technical) Name	*Brand Name(s)*
Amitriptyline	Elavil, Endep, Etrafon, Limbitrol, Triavil
Chlordiazepoxide	Librium, Limbitrol, Menrium
Chlorpromazine	Thorazine
Chlorprothixine	Taractan
Clorazepate dipotassium	Tranxene
Desipramine	Norpramin, Pertofrane
Diazepam	Valium, Valrelease Capsules
Droperidol	Inapsine, Innovar
Fluphenazine	Permitil, Prolixin
Haloperidol	Haldol
Imipramine	Janimine, Tofranil
Isocarboxazide	Marplan
Lithium carbonate	Eslalith, Lithane, Lithobid, Lithonate, Lithotabs
Mesoridazine	Serentil
Meprobamate	Deprol, Equanil, Equagesic, Meprospan, Milpath, Miltown
Nortriptyline	Aventyl, Pamelor
Oxazepam	Serax
Pargylene	Eutonyl
Phenelzine sulfate	Nardil

Drugs for Controlling the Emotions (Tranquilizers, Anti-depressants, Antianxiety Agents)
(Continued)

Generic (Technical) Name	*Brand Name(s)*
Procarbazine hydrochloride	Matulane
Prochloperazine	Combid, Compazine, Prochlor-Iso
Promazine	Sparine
Trifluroperazine	Stelazine
Thioridazine	Mellaril
Thiothixene	Navane
Tranlcypromine sulfate	Parnate
Tybamate	Tybatran

Antihistamines (Treatment of Allergies, Common Cold Preparations, Sleeping Pills, and Motion Sickness Remedies)

Generic (Technical) Name	*Brand Name(s)*
Dimenhydrinate	Dramamine, Nico-Vert
Diphenhydramine	Ambenyl, Benadryl, Benylin, Bromanyl, Dytuss
Hydroxyzine	Vistaril
Meclizine	Antivert, Bonine
Promethazine	Dihydrocodeine Compound Maxigesic, Mepergan Phenergan, Remsed,

Antihistamines (Treatment of Allergies, Common Cold Preparations, Sleeping Pills, and Motion Sickness Remedies)
(Continued)

Generic (Technical) Name   *Brand Name(s)*

Stopayne, Synalgos, Zipan

Drugs for Gastrointestinal Problems (Ulcers, Heartburn, Stomach Pain, Flatulence, and Spastic Colon and Bowels)

Generic (Technical) Name   *Brand Name(s)*

Atropine   Antrocol, Arco-Lase Pills, Butabell, Probocon, Uretron

Propantheline bromide   Pro-Banthine

Cimetidine   Tagamet

Metoclopramide   Regian

Drugs Used for Other Medical Problems[2]

Generic (Technical) Name   *Brand Name(s)*

Acetozolamide (glaucoma)   Diamox

Aminocaproic acid (bleeding)   Amicar

Benztropine (Parkinson's disease)   Cogentin

Biperidin (Parkinson's disease)   Akineton

Drugs Used for Other Medical Problems[2]

(Continued)

Generic (Technical) Name	Brand Name(s)
Cycrimine (Parkinson's disease)	Pagitane
Cyclybenzaprine (muscle spasms)	Flexeril
Indomethacin (arthritis)	Indocin
Levodopa (Parkinson's disease)	Larodopa, Sinemet
Methysergide (severe headaches)	Sansert
Metronidazole (infections)	Flagyl, Satric
Trihexyphenidyl (Parkinson's disease)	Artane
Orphenadrine (muscle spasms)	Norflex, Norgesic, X-Otag
Phenytoin (grand mal seizures)	Dilantin
Procyclidine (Parkinson's disease)	Kemadrin

[1]*Some brand-name drugs appear more than once on list due to more than one active generic ingredient in formulation.*

[2]*Principal use in parentheses.*

Surgery and physical injury

Impotence can result from nerve damage during various types of surgery. This includes surgery for benign enlargement of the prostate; cancer of the prostate, bladder, and rectum; aortic aneurysm resection; and aortal femoral bypass. In the case of radical pelvic surgery for cancer of the prostate, bladder, and rectum, new techniques are now available which are intended to minimize the damage to vital nerve connections. The jury of medical opinion is still out on the effectiveness of such procedures, but the results to date appear encouraging.

Surgical removal of the testicles is sometimes necessitated in cases of cancer of the prostate and in connection with testicular cancer, which is not as common. Impotence is frequently experienced after such surgery.

Impotence can also be caused by nerve damage resulting from accidental damage or trauma. As previously noted, severe injuries to the pelvic region may result in impotence, due to obstructions in the arterial blood vessels supplying the penis. Such injuries may often result in serious nerve damage. Trouble can be expected in approximately one-third of the cases of male pelvic damage.

Spinal cord injuries often result in impotence. The extent of erectile failure, as well as of paralysis throughout the body and other physical problems, depends on the location and severity of the damage. The situation is complicated, but, in general, the less the spinal cord has been severed and the lower down the injury occurs, the better the overall prognosis. When the cord has been only partially severed, erections are still often possible, although in many instances they are of short duration. Injuries at the higher end of the column typically prevent the transmission of erotic thoughts from the brain to the penis to stimulate erections. Such individuals, however, may still have erections of the reflex type with appropriate mechanical stimulation. In treating individuals with spinal cord injuries, efforts to restore sexual function are very important to the patient's overall emotional condition. Research is underway which offers the promise of electrically stimulated ejaculation when such patients want to father children.

Impotence can result, on occasion, from direct physical injury to the penis, either by nerve or blood vessel damage.

Unless the damage has been too severe, function usually returns in time. At times, surgery will be necessitated. An unusual case was that of Tony, age thirty-eight, who injured his penis by falling on a tree stump while deer hunting. The injury resulted in Peyronie's disease, a condition characterized by a seriously bent penis. A surgical procedure was successful in restoring the normal shape of the penis, but a penile implant was eventually required to restore proper sexual function.

Neurological disorders

Various neurological problems can result in impotence. These include both benign and malignant tumors of the brain and spinal cord. Multiple sclerosis, a disease that tends to attack the peripheral regions of the body, resulting in great weakness, often leads to impotence when the nerves serving the penis are damaged. Impotence problems of a neurological nature also may appear in men subject to epilepsy and Parkinson's disease.

PROBLEMS OF BOTH THE BLOOD SUPPLY AND THE NERVOUS SYSTEM

Diabetes

Blood supply and nervous system problems resulting in impotence often occur when a man has diabetes mellitus. Diabetes when untreated, is a potentially life-threatening disease in both men and women. In diabetes, failure of the pancreas to secrete sufficient quantities of the vital substance insulin results in the inability of the body to properly metabolize carbohydrates in the form of sugars and starches. *About one-half of all men in whom diabetes has been detected will typically develop impotence over a ten-year period following the onset of the disease.* Control of diabetes is extremely important through diet and regular visits to your physician.

Diabetes may first occur in childhood or in later life. Juvenile diabetes is generally more serious than adult diabetes, although it can be more rapidly detected and treated. Adult diabetes often develops over a period of time and has less obvious symptoms. Often the first symptom of adult diabetes in men is impotence. For this reason, any man experiencing impotence is well advised to have appropriate urinalysis and blood tests performed to check on the possibility of diabetes. As there is evidence that diabetes involves genetic factors, men with a family history of the disease who experience impotence problems should be especially cautious. Penile fibrosis, a condition in which scar tissue forms within the penis, is also much more common in the diabetic patient.

Vascular disease is believed to represent the most immediate factor causing impotence in diabetic men. Arteriosclerosis, associated with diabetes, results in problems in both the large and small blood vessels of the body, including lesions of the deep penile arteries. The disease, after a period of time, also usually results in serious damage to both the somatic and autonomic nervous systems. Often, matters are complicated in adult male diabetics by obesity and alcoholism.

Kidney disease

In chronic kidney disease, kidney failure often results in abnormal hormone levels which may affect erection. The problems of such patients are often complicated by high blood pressure and the side effects of medications for treating hypertension. There may also be direct damage to nerve circuits leading to the penis.

Kidney failure is life threatening and may require hemodialysis, in which patients must report frequently to treatment centers where they undergo blood filtration using an external artificial kidney. Such treatment is highly stressful and could contribute to pyschological impotence in male patients. There is also reason to suspect that the process may result in chemical changes in the mineral content of the bloodstream that contribute to impotence.

Psychological factors

Psychological factors, acting primarily through the nervous system, may result in impotence, although little is conclusively known about the exact mechanism through which this occurs. The theory, as noted in Chapter 2, that psychological impotence operates through an "adrenalin reflex," may apply best to episodes of temporary impotence, especially in younger men. A sudden rush of adrenalin, of course, occurs in highly fearful situations. Ribald stories about the narrow escape of a young lover, when surprised by an irate husband in *flagrante delicto,* are common to all cultures. The typical story often contains the comic image of the young man leaping from the wife's second-story bedchamber, while simultaneously attempting to pull on a pair of pants (or perhaps adjust a toga). Implicit in such stories is the almost instantaneous loss of erection that occurs under such circumstances.

Fearful situations of this type are uncommon in the case of an older man who gradually experiences chronic impotence after many years of successful sexual perform-ance with a life-long partner. In such cases, it is very reasonable to suspect that causes other than psychological are at the root of the problem.

In summary, many factors can result in impotence. All factors, even those of a strictly psychological nature, must somehow adversely affect the normal functioning of the blood supply and nervous systems. Many of the factors that affect the blood supply are also associated with cardiovascular disease and the aging process. In the case of factors that act through the nervous system, physical injuries, alcohol, drugs, and various neurological disorders can underlie an impotence problem. Finally, the problem is often traced to conditions such as diabetes and kidney disease, which may affect both the blood supply and nervous system.

When to get help — diagnoses that you can do yourself

P rocrastination, unfortunately, is a very common trait in men suffering from sexual dysfunction. In treating impotence, physicians often see individuals who have waited for years before seeking help. And it is a frequent occurrence to hear these patients, overjoyed by their successful treatment, express great regret and even guilt for not having sought help sooner.

Self-recrimination for having procrastinated, however, is not always justified. It is often difficult to know when a problem is serious enough. In individual episodes of impotence, the male partner, of course, is generally quite aware of performance failure. Isolated episodes of impotence, however, are common and do not necessarily show all the signs of being a chronic problem. Just how frequently does failure have to occur before it is reasonable to conclude that help is needed? This is a difficult question to answer. To further complicate the situation, chronic impotence often develops gradually, over a period of years, while the ability to perform may ebb and flow while the overall decline is in progress.

Systematic self-evaluation, combined with reliable background information, is critical in making the decision whether or not to seek help. The objective of this chapter is to provide you with sufficient information to conduct this systematic self-evaluation when various types of male sexual dysfunction are suspected. Major emphasis is given to recognizing the problem of impotence, although the self-evaluation of other dysfunction problems is also included, as well as information on several other male genital problems that are sometimes encountered.

To evaluate your own situation, it is best to keep a simple written record indicating the frequency and extent of performance failure over a period of several months, which you will show to your urologist or health care professional. The availability of a record helps overcome embarrassment when discussing problems with a health care professional. It will also prove helpful if you take along a copy of your answers to the questions shown in the accompanying checklist of possible impotence symptoms.

HOW TO RECOGNIZE IMPOTENCE

An episode of impotence may be said to have occurred when the male partner attempts normal vaginal intercourse and is either unable to achieve an erection of sufficient rigidity for penetration or, given penetration, finds that the duration of the erection proves inadequate for the mutual satisfaction of both parties. Before concluding that impotence has occurred in a given episode, it is sometimes necessary to consider whether the time was sufficient to permit the achievement of an erection and the orgasmic characteristics of the female partner.

The length of time to achieve an erection can vary considerably for different men. A normal man in his mid-

YOUR PERSONAL IMPOTENCE CHECKLIST

Your Current Sexual Performance

1. Have you been experiencing difficulty recently in achieving erections that you and your partner consider adequate for vaginal intercourse?

2. Does this problem occur three out of every four times or more that you attempt intercourse?

3. Is intercourse attempted under what you feel are favorable conditions and with adequate erotic stimulation?

Your Sexual Performance Trends

1. For how long have you been experiencing difficulty in achieving erections?

2. Are morning and spontaneous erections becoming less common?

3. How much longer does it take to achieve erection than in the past?

4. Has it become more difficult to have intercourse in certain sexual positions?

5. Has it become more difficult to successfully masturbate?

Your Medical Condition

1. Have you ever been told you have any form of cardiovascular disease, especially heart disease, arteriosclerosis, peripheral arterial disease (PAD), and/or hypertension?

2. Have you ever had an operation for heart disease or some other cardiovascular problem?

3. Have you ever been told that you have an elevated cholesterol level?

4. Do you ever experience serious pain in the legs when walking?

5. Are you taking any form of drug for a cardiovascular problem, especially hypertension?

6. Are you taking drugs on a prescription basis for any other problem?

7. Do you have any known glandular disorder, especially diabetes?

8. Do you have any known neurological disorder such as multiple sclerosis or epilepsy?

9. Have you ever had major surgery in the pelvic area, especially surgery involving the prostate gland and colon?

10. Have you ever had an injury involving the pelvic area, back, spinal cord, or head?

11. Have you ever been treated with radiation therapy for a problem in the pelvic area?

12. Have you ever had an episode of priapism (persistent longstanding erection)?

Your Personal Life Style

1. Do you now smoke or did you once smoke for a long period of time?

2. Are you a heavy drinker or a diagnosed alcoholic?

3. Have you used various illegal drugs, especially cocaine?

4. Are you a frequent user of nonprescription drugs?

5. Are you excessively overweight?

twenties often experiences an erection in twenty-five seconds given only visual stimulation, such as the presence of an appealing female partner or the viewing of erotic material. Other men, especially with increasing age, tend to require more time and some degree of physical manipulation. It is reasonable to conclude that failure has occurred when an erection is absent after a period of several minutes, assuming a favorable environment, erotic stimulation, and reasonable manipulation by a cooperative partner.

It is more difficult to define how long an erection should be maintained after penetration to allow for the mutual satisfaction of both parties. Loss of an erection, accompanied by ejaculation, during penetration or after the first few pelvic thrusts, constitutes premature ejaculation rather than impotence, and is discussed separately. The maintenance of an erection without desired ejaculation for extended periods, perhaps fifteen minutes or more, is indicative of ejaculatory failure, or retarded ejaculation, and is also discussed separately. Loss of erection prior to ejaculation, either immediately after penetration, or in a relatively short time period, such as five minutes or less, is indicative of impotence.

The length of time an erection should be maintained in order to provide for the satisfaction of the female partner is also a very complex issue. Women differ widely in their ability to achieve orgasm by simple vaginal intercourse. Some women are able to achieve orgasm rapidly in this manner. Other women find it impossible to achieve an orgasm at all by vaginal intercourse. It is unreasonable to conclude that a man is impotent if he is unable to maintain an erection after penetration for a heroic period of time. An erection is adequate, from a male sexual performance standpoint, if it can be sustained within the vagina for a period of about ten minutes. The male, of course, has an obligation to assist his partner in achieving orgasm by other means should this period of time prove to be inadequate. In this connection, it is worth remembering that the fingers never get soft.

The decision to seek professional help for suspected impotence should include a variety of factors. To help make this decision, several simple tests are available that can be performed at home. It is possible that a single factor or physical response to any one test may, by itself, be sufficient to provide a definite indication of a condition requiring professional attention. If this should not be the case, the overall pattern should be considered in making a decision.

Review the pattern of your recent sexual performance

The systematic evaluation of recent sexual performance is the logical starting point in self-evaluation. Recent performance should be examined, and the number of times that episodes of impotence have taken place should be estimated to the best of your ability. In characterizing any given episode as impotence, the preceding discussion of the nature of impotence should be taken into consideration.

Ideally, past performance should be reviewed over a period of several months. Most men, of course, do not normally keep a record of such matters. The analysis, therefore, is inherently subject to a degree of inaccuracy. Involving the female partner may prove useful in improving accuracy.

You can, of course, keep a log of future sexual activity and then analyze the resulting pattern. The problem with this approach is that for some men, the very procedure of keeping a log introduces an element of performance anxiety that could influence the observed pattern.

In general, when impotence occurs one out of every two times, or 50 percent of the time, given a reasonable number of attempts over a period of about a month, there is strong evidence that chronic impotence exists. Under such circumstances, seeking professional assistance is well-justified without any futher analysis. At the level of one out of every four encounters, or 25 percent of the time, there is a strong possibility of a chronic condition. However, you should consider other factors before seeking assistance. A one-out-of-ten failure level, is little reason for immediate concern.

Trends in sexual performance

The tendency for impotence to develop gradually over a period of time, especially in the case of older men, makes it highly advisable to evaluate, as objectively as possible, how your recent sexual behavior compares with that of past years. The onset of impotence very frequently takes place over a two-to-five-year period. During this time, an awareness of the condition gradually emerges. For this reason, going back for a period of about five years is particularly relevant for older men who first become suspicious of a possible impotence condition.

Recalling accurately the frequency of sexual inter-course and the extent of performance failure over a long period of time is very difficult. Fortunately, you can get a good idea of what has been happening by evaluating these three conditions:

- Frequency of morning and spontaneous erections

- Length of time required to initiate and obtain a full erection

- Your ability to assume varied sexual positions

Virtually every healthy young man experiences the presence of a full erection immediately upon awakening from sleep. The presence of such an erection is normal and is related to the frequent erections that occur during sleep.

As a condition of chronic impotence becomes established, the frequency and firmness of morning erections diminish. The total absence of such erections is a strong indication of chronic impotence, usually of a physical origin.

Spontaneous erections occur during waking hours and in the absence of physical stimulation. Such erections are often noticed by younger men when viewing erotic material, or even in casual conversation with attractive women. When spontaneous erections no longer occur in men for whom such erections were previously common, there is a reasonable suggestion of some loss of sexual vigor.

As previously mentioned, with increasing age men usually require more stimulation to achieve erections. Such change can be gradual. A significant change in a relatively short period of time, however, suggests the development of chronic impotence.

A very revealing symptom at the onset of chronic impotence is the increasing inability to assume varied positions during sexual intercourse. Certain men, because of social conditioning or religious beliefs, rarely attempt intercourse in any manner other than the familiar "missionary" position. In the case of a man who has regularly employed different positions, and now finds that intercourse in only one position is possible, there is good indication of an evolving impotence problem, most likely related to changes that have been taking place in the vascular system.

The term "steal syndrome" is used for the type of problem in which erections occur in the resting state, but are rapidly lost after assuming the desired position for intercourse, either immediately following vaginal penetration, or following the first few pelvic thrusts. The term refers to the fact that as the level of sexual activity increases, blood is "stolen" from the penis and pelvic area, resulting in the loss of erection. It may be that the steal syndrome takes place only when certain positions are attempted. Often a change of position, such as the woman on top, may result in improved performance.

Self-evaluation tests you can do at home

Masturbation performance

The ability to masturbate successfully, with a full erection, constitutes a test for chronic impotence that can be easily performed at home. When attempted, there are several possible outcomes:

- There is an absence of both erection and ejaculation.
- Ejaculation takes place in the absence of an erection.
- Both full erection and ejaculation take place.
- Full erection is achieved, but ejaculation does not take place.

When masturbation, performed under suitable conditions, consistently results in neither erection nor ejaculation, chronic impotence of a physical nature is strongly indicated. In Western culture, however, a strong religious and social taboo has historically existed against masturbation. As a consequence, it is possible that some individuals find it virtually impossible to achieve an erection from self-stimulation. In either case, any individual who cannot obtain an erection from self-stimulation, or has no recollection of ever having an erection, is well-advised to seek professional help.

It is quite possible for a man to masturbate to ejaculation despite the absence of an erection, or to ejaculate with an erection of insufficient firmness for vaginal penetration. Chronic impotence is most likely present in such individuals, and professional help should be sought. Because the ability to successfully ejaculate suggests the absence of a psychological barrier against masturbation, it's quite likely that the impotence has physical causes.

When a man who has been experiencing impotence symptoms during sexual intercourse is able to successfully masturbate to ejaculation with a full erection, psychological impotence is a definite possibility. It is possible, however, that the condition has a physical origin. For example, the problem may again be the steal syndrome: the limited physical activities associated with masturbation are not sufficient to result in loss of erection, in contrast with the increased sexual activity that occurs during regular intercourse and results in loss of erection. Regardless of the origin of the problem, professional attention is definitely indicated for men who can successfully masturbate and ejaculate with full erection, but consistently prove impotent during sexual relations with a partner.

The final masturbation possibility, erection without ejaculation, indicates the dysfunction known as ejaculatory failure. An individual who can achieve erection through masturbation, but cannot ejaculate, is usually capable of vaginal penetration.

Postage stamp test

Nocturnal erections occur in periods known as REM (rapid eye movement) sleep, in intervals typically five minutes to one-half hour long, during which dreams usually occur. While in the REM state, it is highly unlikely that psychological factors can prevent erections in a man physically capable of having an erection.

In the professional investigation of impotence, an electronic monitoring instrument is sometimes used to determine the incidence of nocturnal erections. During the test, a sensor is attached to the penis to monitor and record changes in penis size.

It is possible to obtain a reasonable approximation of the test with only a coil of U.S. postage stamps. For economy, use of one-cent stamps is suggested. Prior to retiring for the evening, simply encircle the soft penis with a sufficient number of stamps to form a ring. Moisten the back of one of the end stamps. Overlap the face of the stamp at the other end of the ring and hold the ring in place long enough to stick.

Immediately after awakening the next morning, examine the stamps. If the ring is broken at any one of the perforations, it means that at least one erection did occur during the night. (The postage stamp test, of course, will not reveal whether there has been more than one erection, as can be done with the more complicated medical device.)

If the postage stamp test reveals the absence of a nocturnal erection, there is a very good indication of chronic impotence of a physical origin. If an erection did take place, impotence of a psychological or physical nature is still a possibility.

Simple neurological tests

Three simple tests can be performed at home, by yourself or with a partner, which provide clues to the functioning of the neurological system of the penis and pelvic area. The first, known as the cremasteric reflex test, measures the adequacy of the neural connections to the pelvic area. To perform this test, lie on your back. Then, either you or your partner should make a light quick stroke with a blunt pointed object across several inches of the inner side of your upper thigh. The normal response is a quick upward movement of the testicle on the same side of the body where the stroke was made. The lack of such movement on either side of the body indicates the possibility of a neurological problem in the spinal column or brain. Professional investigation is recommended both for the treatment of impotence as well as for general health.

As all healthy men living outside the tropics know, the scrotum will tighten up and draw upward into the body when exposed to low temperature conditions. This response is part of the normal mechanism used to maintain seminal fluid at the proper temperature for reproductive purposes. In the ice-cube test, an ice cube or some other very cold object is placed momentarily on the scrotum. The normal response should be a rapid, easily observed contraction. Lack of this response indicates a neurological problem warranting professional investigation.

The final test is for the more adventurous, but it can actually be performed easily. The bulbocavernosus, or BC reflex test, involves the insertion of a finger in the anus and the simultaneous quick squeezing of the tip of the penis. If the neurological system is functioning properly, a quick contraction in the rectal area should be felt.

Simple vascular tests

Several simple home tests or observations can be made that provide clues to the possible existence of vascular or blood flow problems possibly related to impotence. The results of these tests or observations are by themselves not conclusive, but they may indicate an overall pattern.

The first is a simple walking test. To perform this test, merely walk a distance of at least one mile at a fairly fast pace. While overexertion should be avoided, the pace and distance should be both faster and somewhat longer than usual. Of course, caution is advised for individuals with known cardiovascular problems. If a fairly piercing pain is noted in either or both calves, evidence exists of an oxygen insufficiency and impaired blood flow to the lower portion of the body. While the walking test does not directly indicate impaired blood flow to the penis, it is a good indication of the possibility.

Examination of the genital area may also yield significant evidence of possible vascular problems. When the penis is found to be consistently cold, even when exposed to warm temperatures, there is a possibility of vascular insufficiency. Abnormalities in the color of the penis are also an important indication of vascular insufficiency. In men with light-colored skin, the penis may take on a distinct blue color when blood flow is impaired. The effect is not as easy to detect with dark-skinned men, but a definite difference in appearance may be noted.

A final observation concerns the presence of firm, hard areas in the penis. Such areas are typically found along both sides of the penis, in the general area where the penis is attached to the body. It is not uncommon to encounter patients at the urologist's office who have noticed hard areas of the penis and are fearful of cancer. Such hard areas, however, usually result from the calcification of the corporal bodies (blood-carrying bodies) in the penis due to the gradual accumulation of plaque. The resulting restriction in blood flow can cause erection difficulties.

Review your medical history

A thorough self-evaluation should include the careful analysis of your personal medical history, particularly with respect to specific health problems known to be linked with impotence. It is especially important to try to relate the onset of any known impotence-linked problem with the first appearance of significant impotence symptoms.

The following list summarizes the most important medical conditions to be considered in self-analysis.

- Cardiovascular diseases
- Diabetes mellitus
- Endocrine (glandular) problems, other than diabetes
- Neurological disorders
- Pelvic surgery
- Accidents to the head, spinal cord, and pelvic area

Men with a history that includes some type of cardiovascular disease should definitely be aware of a possible link with impotence. This is especially true for individuals with heart disease, blood vessel disease, hypertension, or those who have experienced coronary artery bypass surgery. A history of any of these problems, combined with frequent impotence episodes and any possible symptoms observed in the simple vascular tests, strongly indicates the need to seek professional assistance.

Given the strong link between impotence and diabetes, any man with a known case of diabetes should be on the lookout for impotence symptoms, and should be prepared to seek assistance, even if such symptoms have not yet appeared. It is a primary responsibility of any physician treating a diabetes patient to explain the possible sexual ramifications of the disease and to encourage consultation with specialists on sexual dysfunction when indicated. All older men should be on the lookout for possible diabetes symptoms, as the disease often occurs later in life in marginal form and may take a while to be detected. A real warning sign would be a combination of impotence, renal (kidney), and retinal (eye) problems.

Individuals with known glandular disorders should consider the possibility of a connection with any impotence symptoms that are being experienced. Men with known problems of the testicles, particularly those associated with inadequate testosterone production, should be prepared to seek professional attention when impotence symptoms are noted. The same advice applies to men with known problems of the thyroid. When there are no known glandular problems, the presence of extreme obesity, chronic fatigue, and impotence can be an indication that such problems may very well exist.

Neurological disorders are generally believed to be of lesser importance as underlying causes of impotence than cardiovascular disease or diabetes. Men with known nervous system disorders, however, including epilepsy and multiple sclerosis, should be aware of the possible connection, and are advised to seek professional help when experiencing impotence symptoms. Impotence is also linked to various types of brain tumors, which is another good reason not to neglect the presence of persistent impotence symptoms.

Any man who has experienced major surgery in the pelvic region, especially procedures involving the prostate gland and the colon, should seek professional help if impotence symptoms are experienced. Usually, impotence shows up fairly soon after such procedures; however, the onset of the problem can be delayed. Men scheduled for such surgery should always discuss the possibility of impotence in advance with their physician, in the hope that a problem can be avoided or at least minimized.

Individuals who have experienced accidental injuries to the head, spinal cord, and pelvic area are also advised to obtain professional help whenever frequent impotence episodes are noted. It would be helpful to ask the parents or other relatives of a patient about his past injuries or accidents because major childhood injuries, which the patient may have completely forgotten, can be a cause of adult impotence. This can be the case especially with injuries to young boys that took place while in a straddle position, such as when riding a bicycle.

Review your use of prescription and nonprescription drugs

The link between impotence and many frequently used medications is discussed in Chapter 4, along with a listing of many of the problem drugs currently in use today. It is important to recognize that because new drugs are constantly being introduced in the pharmaceutical field, no listing of problem drugs will ever be complete. Therefore, if a drug you are taking or plan to take is not included in the list in Chapter 4, that is no guarantee the drug is free of problems. Fortunately, many newer drugs are much improved with respect to impotence and other side effects, but that is not always the case. If information on any drug that you are taking or will be taking has not been provided by your regular physician, you would be well-advised to consult the latest edition of the *Physicians' Desk Reference,* published annually by Medical Economics Company, Inc., Oradell, New Jersey. This book, commonly known as the "PDR," is usually found at major public libraries. The American Urological Association publishes a listing of drugs linked to sexual dysfunction. The address of this organization, and of several other organizations that provide information on problem drugs is given in Chapter 6.

Any man who has been using a prescription drug linked to impotence should not immediately discontinue its use upon becoming aware of that fact. This sometimes happens, particularly in the case of men using medications for high blood pressure. Such men, of course, subject themselves to the long-term danger of strokes, heart attacks, and other problems. With some drugs, precipitous withdrawal can present a very real immediate danger. The best course of action is to first talk with the physician who has prescribed the suspected drug. Sometimes an alternative medication is available, with lesser side effects. Should your physician be unresponsive, get a second opinion before discontinuing the drug.

Inventory your alcohol and drug use

Any man who is a heavy drinker or a diagnosed alcoholic should be aware of the strong possibility of impotence and should not hesitate to seek help, even when relatively infrequent episodes of impotence are first experienced. Moderate social drinking, however, is not grounds for seeking immediate help, unless an impotence problem is becoming chronic, and other contributory problems are observed in self-evaluation.

Infrequent use of illegal substances, including marijuana and cocaine, in itself is not sufficient reason to conclude that immediate professional attention is required after a few impotence episodes. Heavy users of such substances, however, are advised to seek professional treatment for both impotence and drug dependency, even after a relatively small number of impotence episodes.

As discussed, smoking tobacco tends to decrease the flow of blood throughout the vascular system, and specifically in the penile artery. Cigarette smokers experiencing symptoms should consider trying the simple vascular tests described previously. If these tests reveal the possible presence of a vascular problem, it would be a good idea to obtain help even after a relatively small number of impotence episodes.

HOW TO RECOGNIZE SEXUAL DYSFUNCTION PROBLEMS OTHER THAN IMPOTENCE

The accompanying table provides a summary of male dysfunction problems. The common definitions shown in the table should prove useful in clearly stating the nature of your problem, should the need for help be indicated. Of course, it is possible to experience a combination of dysfunction problems.

SUMMARY OF MALE SEXUAL DYSFUNCTION PROBLEMS

Problem	Common Definition
Impotence	The inability to achieve an erection of sufficient rigidity for vaginal penetration, or of sufficient duration for the mutual satisfaction of both partners.
Premature Ejaculation	Ejaculation that takes place well before the time desired by both sexual partners.

Problem	Common Definition
Retrograde Ejaculation	Ejaculation usually taking place with adaquate physical sensation, but without the normal flow of ejaculatory fluid from the tip of the penis. The fluid backs up into the bladder and subsequently passes harmlessly out of the body during normal urination.
Ejaculatory Failure	The inability to ejaculate within a reasonable period of time or not at all, despite the ability to achieve and maintain an adequate erection.
Priapism	Painful and unwanted erections that continue for extended periods of time.
Peyronie's Disease	A condition characterized by a penis that is bent out of shape during erection and often subject to pain and discomfort.
Painful Ejaculation	Pain or abnormal discomfort experienced during ejaculation.
Lack of Desire	The complete or nearly complete abnormal absence of sexual interest (libido).
Performance Anxiety	The abnormal fear of engaging in sexual activities.

Premature ejaculation

Ejaculation that frequently takes place well before it is desired by either sexual partner is considered premature. Some men with the problem will ejaculate spontaneously during foreplay, or very shortly after first being touched in the genital area. Most men with the problem, however, ejaculate during vaginal penetration, but after only the first few pelvic thrusts.

It is a popular belief that premature ejaculation is almost always a problem experienced by sexually naive younger men in early sexual encounters. The extraordinary level of arousal that is supposed to occur under such circumstances presumably causes almost instantaneous erection and ejaculation. Mild versions of the supposedly comical and usually humiliating event have on occasion been portrayed on the stage and screen.

Jeff, a thirty-eight-year-old financial executive, began to experience premature ejaculation with his wife after fifteen years of marriage. His problem was complicated by guilt over a recent extramarital affair. He reasoned that his problem was somehow due to an excess of ardor brought on by a need to compensate for his feelings of guilt.

While premature ejaculation may have a psychological cause, it can also have a physical origin. The problem may frequently occur in men with infections of the prostate. In such cases, the problem usually makes its appearance shortly after the onset of the infection. Examination revealed that Jeff had an inflamed prostate. The premature ejaculation condition disappeared after treatment. The link between premature ejaculation and prostate infections makes it logical to regard premature ejaculation as a possible symptom of a prostate infection.

To determine if a premature ejaculation problem exists, you should first record how often you have experienced the symptom. As with impotence, a period of at least one month should be examined. It is reasonable to seek professional help when the problem occurs during approximately one out of every four sexual encounters, or about 25 percent of the time.

Before seeking help, it would be a good idea to examine yourself for indications of an inflamed prostate. These include:

- A penile discharge of a generally white appearance

- Ejaculate which appears bloody

- Burning sensation when urinating

- Unusually frequent urination at night

- Restricted flow during urination and frequent stopping and starting of the urinary stream during urination

The simple examination of the prostate that is typically performed in a routine physical examination is generally not enough to diagnose a prostatic infection capable of causing premature ejaculation. A vigorous massage of the prostate by a urological specialist and the laboratory examination of expelled prostatic fluid are required.

Retrograde ejaculation

In retrograde ejaculation, there is no flow of ejaculatory fluid from the tip of the penis. Although retrograde ejaculation does not normally reduce the sexual pleasure to either partner, it is an obvious problem when children are desired. The condition occurs when the sphincter muscle that usually shuts off the passageway through which urine travels from the bladder to the penis during periods of sexual activity fails to function properly. When this happens, ejaculatory fluid backs up into the bladder. Subsequently, the fluid passes harmlessly out of the body during normal urination.

Damage to the sphincter can be caused by routine prostate surgery, damage to the nerves at the base of the bladder, and spinal cord injury. Another cause is diabetes and for this reason, especially, the condition should not be neglected.

It may be some time before the existence of a retrograde ejaculation problem is observed, as the feeling of ejaculation continues even in the absence of ejaculate. A slight cloudy condition seen in the first urination following intercourse may be the first symptom. Should this be seen, it is, of course, possible to check for the presence of ejaculate in the vagina of the partner. The absence of ejaculate in the vagina, however, is not always obvious. Masturbation represents the conclusive test for the condition.

Ejaculatory failure

Ejaculatory failure, or the failure to ejaculate, is fortunately a relatively rare condition, as it is difficult to treat. The cause of the problem has yet to be satisfactorily determined, but there is evidence that both psychological and physical factors may play a role.

Masters and Johnson studies have suggested that the problem is largely psychological, and occurs most often in men with very sexually inhibiting religious and moral backgrounds. Theresa Larsen Crenshaw, M.D., a sex therapist based in southern California, has observed that the overwhelming number of men who report the problem are from Jewish backgrounds. This has not always been found to be the case however. In Atlanta, a metropolitan area with a relatively low Jewish population, ejaculatory failure shows up as frequently in patients as elsewhere.

If ejaculatory failure were to be demonstrated to be a problem highly characteristic of Jewish men, one possible explanation might be cultural attitudes that result in psychological barriers to sexual performance. Inhibiting attitudes toward sexual matters exist among traditional Jews, as in most traditional cultures. This does not seem to have prevented the existence of the very large families characteristic of the fundamentalist sect known as the Hasidim.

Another explanation might be the religious practice of circumcision common to both the Jewish and Islamic traditions. Circumcision does somewhat decrease the sensitivity of the tip of the penis, with conceivable psychological or physical consequences. The problem with this explanation is that most American men have been routinely circumcised since the 1940s. At present, about 80 percent of all American males are circumcised, although the operation is rarely a medical necessity. If circumcision was the root cause of ejaculatory failure, the problem would obviously be far more common. The consistent inability to ejaculate within a period of fifteen minutes or even more, despite the presence of a firm erection and suitable surroundings, is indicative of ejaculatory failure. When failure occurs 25 percent of the time or more, professional help is indicated.

When the problem is experienced with one partner, but not another, or when the man subject to the problem is able to successfully masturbate, it is reasonable to assume that psychological factors are at work. The presence of the problem, combined with the inability to successfully masturbate, tends to indicate an increased likelihood of a physical problem, although this is not always the case.

Priapism

Priapism derives its name from the minor Greek god, Priapus. The deity was portrayed in antiquity by a figure with an enormous, constantly erect phallus (penis). Despite the many tall tales told by "studs," supererections that last for hours are not an everyday occurrence, or anything to be admired.

Priapism is a serious condition that should receive immediate medical attention, regardless of any embarrassment. The danger is that the extended interruption of the supply of oxygen and other constituents of the blood to the penis that occurs in priapism can result in extensive internal damage to the penis rendering the normal erection mechanism inoperative.

During an incident of priapism, the blood becomes sludge-like, a condition that can directly cause impotence, due to the blockage of blood flow. The condition can occur in cancer. Also, an erection suggestive of priapism may occur during injection therapy, when the drug papaverine is being used to promote erection.

Distinguishing an erection due to priapism from a normal erection is usually not too difficult. Any erection that persists without continuing physical stimulation, for more than one-half hour, and is not relieved through ejaculation or negative thought processes, is suspect, unless erections of this duration have been common in the past. In priapism, erections can actually last for several days, but help should be obtained after an unwanted erection continues for more than several hours. Erections obtained by the use of the drug papaverine in an impotence treatment program under a urologist's direction normally last one to two hours. Chapter 7 discusses what to expect and what you should do in this type of treatment.

Peyronie's disease

Peyronie's disease, or the bent penis syndrome, is caused by the formation of scar tissue along the walls of the erectile chambers of the penis. This scarring results from plaque deposits and, in time, results in the bending of the penis in the direction of the side of the penis where the scarring is most severe.

Peyronie's disease often occurs, without any obvious reason, in men age forty and older. The disease sometime occurs in men who are heavy users of alcohol. At times, the symptoms of the disease disappear on their own. In almost one-third of the cases, the disease results in significant penile deformity and painful erection. In some cases, an erection may occur at the rear of the penis, beyond the point of maximum plaque buildup, but not at the front or downstream end. Often, the deformity and pain it causes during erection may be sufficient to make vaginal penetration difficult, if not impossible.

Peyronie's disease should be suspected and help obtained whenever there has been a noticeable change in the shape of the erect penis. The condition usually develops over a period of time, and is often overlooked until painful erection makes vaginal penetration difficult.

Just as women are advised to perform periodic breast self-examination, it is a good idea for all men to regularly check the general condition of their penis and testicles. A sign of possible Peyronie's disease is a buildup of scar tissue that can be felt beneath the skin of a nonerect penis. In examining the testicles, it is important to check for any change in size, or any change that may be felt inside the scrotum.

Painful ejaculation

The sensations of pleasure and pain are, to a degree, interconnected in brain and nervous system. As a consequence, it may be difficult to distinguish low levels of pain from pleasure during ejaculation. The difficulty is compounded by the obvious preoccupation of the man during sexual intercourse. At more intense levels of discomfort, however, a painful condition should become quite obvious. Painful ejaculation can actually extend to a point where sexual activities are precluded.

There are various causes of painful ejaculation. The most common problem is an infection of the prostate and/or one or both of the seminal vesicles. If there is any doubt that pain is being felt, masturbation represents a good way to check. Persistent pain should be investigated professionally, especially if other symptoms are apparent, such as unusual penile discharges.

Lack of desire

Sexual interest, or libido, is a very normal characteristic of all healthy males beyond the age of puberty. Sexual interest, of course, is held in check by social convention, moral convictions, and the legal system. The lack of sexual desire, even in an individual who, for religious purposes, has taken a vow of chastity, is abnormal, and may be symptomatic of an underlying physical problem. In the marital situation, lack of desire can often weaken or damage the marital relationship.

Possible physical causes of lack of desire include hyperthyroidism and kidney problems. Anything, such as alcoholism, that depresses testosterone or increases estrogen production, can result in lack of desire.

Men with a lack of sexual desire are not always aware of the condition. Often the matter is first mentioned by the partner. If lack of desire becomes apparent in a stable relationship between two partners, it is helpful to observe whether certain physical conditions often associated with lack of desire are apparent, such as chronic fatigue, general malaise, and depression. Such symptoms may indicate hyperthyroidism. It is also advisable to investigate any change that may be noticed in the size and shape of the testicles, allowing for the possibility of some impairment in testosterone production. Professional help should be obtained whenever lack of desire persists for several months or is combined with the other symptoms noted previously.

Performance anxiety

Performance anxiety is characterized by the abnormal fear of sexual activities in a man whose libido remains at normal levels. A man experiencing this condition may consciously or unconsciously avoid contact with potential sexual partners or avoid sexual relations with an existing partner.

In the past, performance anxiety has generally been considered essentially a psychological problem caused by such factors as guilt, fear of punishment, and fear of possible ridicule by a sexual partner. As noted in Chapter 1, the popular belief that the feminist movement, characterized by more sexually aware and demanding women, has resulted in the increased incidence of performance anxiety problems in men, is not supported by scientific evidence.

Psychological explanations of performance anxiety do not adequately account for problems of this nature that may arise in older men, who have successfully engaged in sexual activities for many years, typically with a long-time partner. In such cases, the underlying cause of performance anxiety may be the onset of impotence brought on by one or more very real physical problems. Performance anxiety problems may be triggered in some men by premature ejaculation resulting from a physical cause.

Performance anxiety is easily detected when obvious symptoms such as panic, fear, increased pulse rate, and hyperventilation take place before and during a sexual situation. The problem is more difficult to detect in a man who unconsciously avoids sexual contacts. The persistence of obvious symptoms indicates a need for professional help. Adult males who are aware of a strong desire for sex, but deliberately avoid the sexual act, should also seek assistance. This, of course, does not apply to men who are obligated or required to be celibate.

HOW TO RECOGNIZE OTHER MALE URINARY-GENITAL SYSTEM PROBLEMS

There are a number of other problems that can affect the male urinary-genital system. While these do not always have immediate implications with respect to successful sexual performance, they should not be ignored due to their general health consequences and possible contribution to a dysfunction problem in the long term. In some cases, these problems may also compromise the health of the partner.

Blood in the urine

Blood in the urine is a serious symptom that deserves prompt professional attention. This advice applies equally to men and women. Possible underlying problems of a serious nature include kidney and bladder tumors. Less serious problems may include various bacterial or viral infections of the bladder, kidney, and urethra.

Detecting blood in the urine is usually not difficult. At times, urine can take on an unusual color that may be mistaken for blood, due to the presence of dyes originating in the diet or in medications. For example, urine may take on an orange-red color after taking Azo-Gantrisin and Pyridium. If there is any doubt in such a situation, it is best to promptly seek professional attention. Small quantities of blood in the urine are difficult to detect visually, but do show up in standard urinalysis procedures.

Penile discharges

Any unusual penile discharge should be investigated. A whitish discharge, not ejaculate, generally indicates urethritis or a prostate infection. In the former category, chlamydia infections are the most common today. Bloody ejaculate usually results from a prostate infection.

A yellowish discharge, usually accompanied by a burning sensation and frequent urination, can indicate gonorrhea, although other causes are possible. Men noticing this symptom have an obvious responsibility to discontinue sexual activity and to advise sexual partners of the possibility of a problem.

Penile skin disorders

Any unusual condition on the skin of the penis that persists for more than a few days deserves professional attention. This includes sores, lumps, and encrusted deposits. In all cases, it is advisable to discontinue sexual activity until the problem is resolved.

Sores and lumps on the penis can indicate various sexually transmitted diseases, such as syphilis and genital herpes. Encrusted deposits may be linked to sexual activities with a partner subject to certain types of vaginitis. When genital herpes proves to be the problem, future sexual activity is possible, but should take place only under suitable circumstances. Intercourse is generally safe during periods when sores are not active in either partner. When a vaginal infection is discovered in the female partner, intercourse should be discontinued until the problem is treated in both partners. Unless this is done, the possibility exists of passing the infection back and forth indefinitely.

Painful urination

Painful urination, similar to painful ejaculation, may indicate a prostate infection. Painful urination may also indicate kidney stones or tumors in the urinary system. All persistent pain should be investigated. Excessive or frequent urination, often accompanied by excessive thirst, can be a symptom of diabetes. This symptom can also occur in certain types of bladder infections.

Knowing when to get help for a suspected male sexual dysfunction problem requires systematic self-evaluation.

After conscientiously applying the information provided in this chapter, you should be able to discern whether or not you have an impotence problem or some other dysfunctional condition of sufficient seriousness to require professional attention. If you determine that you do not need professional help, your effort will still have been worthwhile, in view of what you have learned about the functioning of your body. You will also be prepared for what may develop in the future.

Should you need professional help, the next chapter, on sources of help, will be of immediate assistance. The information you accumulated in your self-evaluation, especially if recorded on paper, is the type of information you will need to discuss your condition intelligently with a physician.

CHAPTER 6

Where to get help — and what to expect

You have carefully followed the suggestions of the previous chapter and have reason to believe that some physical problems exist. You are now faced with a major problem: finding effective help. If you live in a typical large urban center, you are faced with making an essentially uninformed choice between a large number of individual health care providers. Unfortunately, few communities enjoy an efficient referral system for finding a suitable physician. You should be concerned about the degree of understanding and professional capability of any practitioner selected at random from the telephone book. Normally, in seeking a physician, you would ask the advice of friends and acquaintances. But understandably, many people are reluctant to do this when the problem is a sexual dysfunction.

This chapter is intended to provide you with a systematic approach to obtaining help. It will also tell you what you should expect and where things can go wrong.

The logical place to start, even if your self-evaluation suggests your problem is psychological in nature, is with a physician familiar with the physical causes of impotence and other male sexual problems. Given the current state of the art, there is virtually no objective way to make a direct diagnosis of psychological impotence. Basically, it is not possible to conclude that psychological impotence exists until all symptoms and known medical problems associated with physical impotence are shown conclusively, by physical examination, not to be present. Failure to eliminate physical impotence as a possibility could result in costly and fruitless psychological treatment or sex therapy. The danger also exists that a potentially dangerous physical problem could go undetected for an extended period.

HOW YOUR REGULAR PHYSICIAN CAN HELP YOU

If a truly efficient system for the delivery of medical services existed, all of us would have convenient and continuing access to a personal physician. Such a physician would be a highly experienced generalist, with a working knowledge of all aspects of medicine and an ongoing familiarity with the medical background of all regular patients. The physician would not be expected to be an expert in every area of medical specialization, but rather an expert on screening medical problems and on preliminary diagnosis. The physician would also be in a position to rapidly access computerized data bases containing the very latest medical information merely by inputting a desktop computer terminal connected electronically to all major world medical centers. When preliminary diagnosis indicated the need for specialized follow-up treatment, the physician, most likely using a computer, would have the capability of providing the patient with the most appropriate referral.

Unfortunately, this ideal of systematic medical practice does not yet exist. Many individuals, however, do have an established relationship with a physician, perhaps a specialist in family medicine, an internist, or a cardiologist. This physician offers the advantage of at least knowing something about the patient's medical history. Typically, men faced with problems of sexual dysfunction initially consult this physician. In the case of subscribers to health maintenance organizations (HMOs) or members of many group care health plans, there is usually no choice other than to contact a physician affiliated with the plan. This physician is often known as your "primary health care provider," or some similar designation.

What you should expect from your physician

It is unreasonable to expect your regular physician to be an authority on male sexual problems. On the other hand, you are entitled, at the very least, to the following when consulting your physician:

- Your problem should be received with understanding and concern. You should receive a full hearing, and under no circumstance should the importance of the problem be minimized. Your physician should make every effort to be reassuring, to put you at ease, and to help you in the difficult task of expressing your problem.

- A careful review should be made of your medical record, and your physician should give special attention to any history of high blood pressure, cardiovascular disease, diabetes, and other physical conditions and life-style problems, such as excessive alcohol intake, associated with male sexual dysfunction. Where indicated, the medical record should be supplemented with additional relevant tests.

- Your physician should review in detail the known adverse reactions of all medications that you are currently taking. If necessary, the physician should contact the indicated pharmaceutical manufacturers and professional colleagues for more complete information on possible side effects. Particular attention should be paid to drugs used in the treatment of high blood pressure. Where medically prudent, the physician should have no objection to prescribing alternative medications with possibly less serious side effects.

● Should a condition that is strongly linked with sexual dysfunction be found, your physician should be prepared to immediately refer you to a urologist specializing in male sexual problems. If there is reason to believe that your condition is due to prescription drugs or life-style problems, the physician should make appropriate recommendations and then carefully track the results over a reasonable period of time. If no change is then noted in your problem, the physician should be prepared to make a prompt referral.

What can go wrong

The following summarizes the experiences of Mort, a fifty-nine-year-old patient:

> At age thirty-five, the patient learned during a routine physical examination that he had moderately elevated blood pressure. His physician, an internist, prescribed an antihypertensive medication containing a diuretic and a tranquilizer. He did not warn the patient of the possible effect on sexual performance. Subsequently, the patient began to experience occasional episodes of impotence, which he told his doctor about during an office visit. In response, the physician stated that impotence was "almost always" psychological in origin, and thus terminated the discussion.

> About five years later, the patient, now living overseas, experienced some pain while urinating

and consulted a local urologist. The problem, traced to a prostate infection, was easily cured. In the course of treatment, the urologist warned of the possible adverse side effects of the patient's high blood pressure medication. The patient followed the urologist's advice, successfully controlled the hypertension problem through weight reduction, and discontinued the medication. The episodes of impotence became very infrequent.

Returning from overseas, the patient was thrown into a high-stress executive position. Given the all-too-frequent combination of stress and unavoidable business entertaining, the patient, in time, was again significantly overweight. The patient, now age fifty, had occasion to consult a physician regarding a gastrointestinal problem. The physician, a gastroenterologist, observing high blood pressure, insisted that the patient resume taking antihypertensives. This time, preparations of both the diuretic and beta-blocker type were prescribed. Again, no warning was volunteered as to possible side effects. In a relatively short time, the patient was again experiencing impotence episodes. When the patient complained about this problem, he was told by the physician that impotence is a normal consequence of aging, and that he should not worry about it. The physician then changed the conversation to a discussion of the importance of an annual proctological examination. The patient's further attempts to bring up the subject of impotence proved futile.

Variations on the preceding story are heard almost daily by urologists specializing in male sexual dysfunction. Unfortunately, all too many physicians are still embarrassed by the subject, or are fundamentally unsympathetic to the problem. Even when true concern exists, the physician may be poorly informed on the subject, and too quick to attribute the patient's condition to psychological problems or aging.

Under no circumstances should you let your physician convince you that you are too old for sexual activities. In fact, if he or she attempts to do so, it is a good idea to get another physician, as such an opinion could indicate a practitioner who is uninformed on modern medical developments in general. It is worth noting that a penile implant is enabling a ninety-five-year-old patient to enjoy a successful sex life.

Some special problems

The increasing importance of group medical programs creates special problems for individuals seeking assistance. As mentioned, a subscriber to an HMO has no choice but to bring a problem of male sexual dysfunction initially to an HMO-designated physician. This physician can prove to be unsympathetic, unknowledgeable, or both. Moreover, such physicians are typically under pressure to minimize referrals to specialists, as a means of controlling costs. Under such circumstances, the subscriber must aggressively pursue the matter with the designated physician, or insist that another physician be appointed under the plan. In extreme cases, there is little choice but to shift to an alternative medical program.

A problem can also exist in dealing with physicians in group medical practice. Group practice, in which perhaps a dozen physicians with different medical specialties join forces in a single corporate entity, and share physical facilities, accounting services, and so forth is the fastest growing segment of the medical profession. The growth of group practice is strongly stimulated by current underlying economic trends impacting on medical practice. In consulting a group practice, you should take into consideration the reasonable likelihood that an attempt will be made to refer all male sexual problems to group members. This could be a problem when no member of the group has a strong capability in treating dysfunction.

Special problems also exist for individuals locked into medical programs based upon a specific employer. An example would be a member of the U. S. armed forces. Individuals enrolled in such programs can face problems, both with respect to obtaining capable medical attention, and with respect to confidentiality. Preserving confidentiality could have important career implications. In some instances, there may be little choice but to seek specialized treatment on a private basis.

Finally, given the highly mobile U.S. population and other factors, many men do not have a regular physician. In such cases, it is reasonable to start directly with a urologist specializing in dysfunction. Various support groups and information services mentioned later in this chapter can prove useful in this connection.

THE ROLE OF THE UROLOGIST SPECIALIZING IN MALE DYSFUNCTION

Urologists are licensed physicians specializing in the treatment of problems of the urinary or urogenital tract. These include such problems as kidney and bladder disorders. As such, a urologist may treat both men and women. In recent years, the role of urologists in the treatment of "male trouble" has grown in importance. In many respects, urologists are assuming a role in the treatment of men parallel to that of gynecologists who treat "female trouble."

Until recently, the treatment by urologists of problems unique to men concentrated on such problems as prostate disorders, testicular disease, and conditions specific to the male urinary tract. In view of the belated attention given to male sexual dysfunction, many excellent practicing urologists still do not enjoy strong capabilities in this area. This should be taken into consideration when seeking help.

What you should expect from your urologist

Unless your condition is especially complicated, a urologist specializing in male sexual dysfunction should be able to determine in two or three visits whether there are specific physical causes underlying your impotence or other dysfunction problem. At least two visits are required before a positive treatment program can be recommended, because of the need to evaluate several important laboratory tests.

On the initial visit, you can expect the following:

- A lengthy and detailed discussion with the urologist
- A detailed physical examination
- The taking of blood, urine, and prostate fluid samples for laboratory analysis

The initial discussion typically covers a review of dysfunction symptoms and past medical history. You will also be questioned as to your pattern of personal relationships, family and job related stress, and similar matters that may have possible psychological implications.

The physical examination includes an inspection for abnormalities throughout the entire genital region, as well as observations and tests to provide evidence of any vascular, neurological, and hormonal difficulty. Inspection of the penis includes checking for scarring, Peyronie's disease, or any abnormal opening of the urethra. An examination is made of the prostate, and a sample of prostate fluid is obtained for examination. The vascular investigation includes the measurement of blood pressure of the penis, using a sonic probe device based upon a principle of physics known as the Doppler effect. Whenever penile blood pressure is found to be 65 percent or less of the normal arm blood pressure measurement, the possibility exists of insufficient blood supply to the penis. Finally the urologist will perform a series of tests to examine the key neurological reflexes in the genital area.

The subsequent laboratory analysis of body fluids is largely to determine the possibility of diabetes and hormonal problems, in particular abnormally low testosterone and abnormally high prolactin levels. A test to determine thyroid activity may also be run using the blood sample.

Tests the urologist administers

Depending on the circumstances, the following additional tests may be performed during subsequent visits.

Nocturnal penile tumescence monitoring (NPT)

Nocturnal penile tumescence monitoring, performed under medical direction, represents an advanced version of the simple home postage stamp test discussed in Chapter 5. NPT monitors vary in design and capabilities, depending upon the manufacturer. All monitors incorporate sensor mechanisms that are placed around the base and near the tip of the penis, permitting the continuous monitoring and recording of all changes that may occur in penile dimensions during REM sleep. Examination of the hard copy produced by the monitor will reveal whether erectile activity has taken place. The result is considered positive when simultaneous expansion is noted at the base and tip of the penis. The newest, most sophisticated monitors also incorporate the capability to measure the rigidity of the penis, and thus provide a further indication of the potential ability to achieve normal vaginal penetration.

Depending upon the degree of accuracy required, NPT testing may be carried out at home, in the urologist's office, or in a hospital sleep laboratory. In sleep lab testing, more sophisticated equipment is used, and attendants are available to check on the equipment, to observe and grade penile rigidity, and sometimes to photograph erections. In some labs, the brain waves of patients are also monitored by EEG devices, to determine the mode of sleep.

It is obvious that overnight testing in a sleep lab is an expensive proposition compared to office testing or testing at home using a portable NPT. It is also far less convenient and more stressful to the patient. Such testing, however, can be required by some insurance carriers. Other carriers may accept testing done in physicians' offices or at home, or not require NPT testing at all. While NPT testing can provide useful results, many urologists do not routinely perform the tests, harboring reservations as to cost-effectiveness. Such urologists reason that adequate tools exist at less cost to the patient, including a simple test that can be performed overnight at home.

It is important to be aware that the presence of an erection at night is not definite evidence of the ability to perform normal sexual activities. This should be kept in mind in dealing with an insurance company that relies heavily on NPT results in determining coverage of treatment.

Papaverine stimulated erection test

The use of the drug papaverine in the treatment of impotence is discussed in Chapter 7. The drug, however, is useful in diagnosis. In the test, a small quantity of the drug is injected directly into the penis. When an erection does not take place shortly, it indicates the possibility of a serious blockage in the arterial system blood supply to the penis or a leak in the downstream venous blood system, which could result in a failure to entrap or maintain blood in the corpora cavernosa when stimulus for an erection exists.

Arteriography

When there is reason to suspect that blockage of the arterial blood supply to the penis may underlie an impotence problem, it is possible to check with an arteriograph test.

There are variations in test methods, but all involve the injection of a harmless solution into an upstream point in the arterial system. The injected solution moves downstream into the key blood vessels that supply the penis. As this takes place, X-ray photographs are taken at various angles of the pelvic area. The injected solution serves as a photographic contrast medium and permits the urologist examining the developed plates to determine the location and extent of any area of blockage. In some instances, the test may be performed with the penis in a state of erection induced by papaverine.

Corpora cavernosagram

The taking of a corpora cavernosagram can be helpful in evaluating damage to the penis from Peyronie's disease, in detecting impotence possibly caused by leaking veins within the corpora cavernosa structure of the penis, or in treating a priapism episode. The test involves the injection of a photographic contrasting fluid into the penis, followed by a series of X-rays. Measurements of blood pressure within the corpora cavernosa may be taken during the procedure. Some procedures may also involve stimulation of an erection, and the taking of penile dimensions as the test proceeds.

Nerve conduction tests

Nerve conduction tests are used to determine the effectiveness of the nerve pathways employed for erection in the conducting of electrical impulses. In the test procedure, electrodes are used to measure electrical characteristics associated with the bulbocavernosus reflex. An analogy exists with circuit testing procedures commonly used by electrical and electronic technicians in spotting circuit problems. When the bulbocavernosus reflex latency time is found to be abnormally long, there is an indication that some neurological problem may underlie impotence.

When all necessary tests have been completed, the urologist will be in a position to provide a diagnosis of the problem and make specific recommendations. Possibilities could include drug or hormonal therapy, the surgical correction of vascular problems, or a penile implant. Referrals to other medical specialists may be appropriate when the impotence problem is found to be symptomatic of a medical condition such as diabetes. If no evidence of a physical cause can be found, referral to a sex therapist may be in order.

Most problems that arise with urologists who specialize in male sexual dysfunction usually involve unreasonable patient expectations. Brad, a forty-five-year-old recovered alcoholic, objected to the advice that a penile implant was the only effective solution to his problem. He was convinced that there was a miracle drug or operative procedure that could repair the permanent physical damage to his body caused by alcoholism. Ronald, age fifty, was disappointed with the results of his implant. It had restored his sexual function, but it did not solve his other problem, a foundering personal relationship with his partner. Patients and partners, therefore, are advised to fully communicate their expectations to their urologist and to carefully understand the implications of the resulting advice.

THE ROLE OF PSYCHOTHERAPISTS
AND SEX THERAPISTS

It is very important to recognize that individuals calling themselves psychotherapists, sex therapists, or some similar term can differ widely as to education and training, surveillance of their professional activities by governmental or professional bodies, and treatment approaches. Individuals offering services related to male sexual dysfunction include psychiatrists, psychologists, social workers, religious counselors, hypnotists, and many others. Psychiatrists, of course, are licensed physicians with medical degrees. The educational credentials of others can range from no university degree to Ph.D.s.

Treatment approaches are also highly varied. In general, individuals calling themselves sex therapists tend to emphasize psychological conditioning techniques rooted in contemporary behavioral psychology theory. Psychological counselors, on the other hand, tend toward more conventional one-on-one or group therapy sessions. The former tend to attack the sexual problem directly, while the latter tend to explore broader aspects of the patient's background.

Many highly competent and reputable individuals are available for sex therapy or psychological counseling on sexual problems. The field, however, is subjective and, at this stage of knowledge, it is more of an art than a science. Under these circumstances, it is not possible for governmental or professional regulation to fully protect the public from the ever-present possibility of quackery. In seeking treatment, therefore, it is wise to follow your urologist's referral. It is also advisable to contact a sex therapist or counselor affiliated with an accredited university or major medical center.

What you should expect from your psychotherapist or sex therapist

A discussion of the important specific treatment approaches used by psychotherapists and sex therapists appears in Chapter 9. The following summarizes what you are entitled to, in a general sense, when consulting such practitioners:

- Your therapist should request and review any

information provided by your urologist or other relevant medical records.

- You should have ample opportunity to discuss the nature of your problem in detail at an extended initial meeting. At this interview, the therapist should not hesitate to provide information on professional credentials and qualifications relevant to treating problems similar to yours.

- You should be provided at the initial meeting, or soon thereafter, with a general appraisal of your problem and treatment prospects. A reputable therapist will not promise a miracle, but will offer an objective assessment of the probability of success based upon the information on hand regarding your individual circumstances and results observed in treating similar patients.

- Prior to the actual commencement of treatment, you should be fully informed as to the methods used in the treatment program. This should include specific information as to what will occur at treatment sessions; the length and frequency of sessions, and the degree of involvement, if any, of your partner. Anything unusual or possibly objectionable in the treatment program (for example, the possible use of female sexual surrogates), should be made abundantly clear and agreed upon well in advance of the start of treatment. Any possible choices between alternative treatment approaches should also be made available at this time.

- While it is understood that it may be initially difficult to determine how long the treatment program will take, you should, nevertheless, be given a preliminary estimate of treatment duration and a full disclosure of associated costs.

- Throughout the entire program, the therapist should

deal with you on a sympathetic and nonjudgmental basis. There should be a willingness to discuss your progress at any time during the program and, if indicated, to alter the treatment approach or terminate the program. There should also be a willingness to involve your urologist or other medical advisor in the program on a continuing and co-operative basis.

What can go wrong

Despite the occasional, possibly lurid, horror story appearing in the popular media as to what may happen to individuals when they consult psychotherapists and sex therapists, the most common problem is the expenditure of considerable sums of money for lengthy and ineffective treatment. Robert had been unable to consummate his relationship with his wife at any time over a period of seventeen years. Over the period, both Robert and his wife had undergone intensive psychotherapy. Robert had been told that his problem was due to repressed sexual feelings toward his mother. When Robert turned up at a urologist's office, a simple test of prolactin level revealed a reading of 180 units, as compared to the normal level of 11. Robert's problem, all along, was caused by a pituitary tumor. The advanced stage of Robert's tumor indicated that the problem causing impotence could have been detected years earlier.

The possibility of losing valuable time and money is greatest when undertaking traditional psychoanalytical treatment, which is by nature open-ended, as compared to the more structured approaches used in the sex therapy of the Masters and Johnson type. It should be noted that most proponents of traditional psychoanalysis do not attempt to hide the fact that treatment will be lengthy, sometimes arguing that it can take several years before sufficient rapport can be established to actually achieve results. Therefore, before you start any sex therapy, first check for the possible existence of a physical problem.

Episodes of victimization by therapists, involving some form of sexual exploitation of the patient, do occur from time to time. Most such situations, however, are believed to involve female, rather than male patients, and, accordingly, are probably not often encountered by men being treated for sexual dysfunction.

SUPPORT GROUPS AND INFORMATION SERVICES

In recent years, a number of support and counseling groups concerned with male sexual dysfunction have been established. A list of such groups, and other organizations providing useful information on a national and sometimes international basis, is provided in this chapter. Many local hospitals hold Impotents Anonymous meetings or meetings of similar organizations.

Impotents Anonymous (I.A.), probably the largest support group, dates to about 1981. The functions and activities of the organization have significant similarities with older support groups such as Alcoholics Anonymous. Local I.A. chapters are affiliated with the Impotence Institute of America, Maryville, Tennessee, a nonprofit educational and charitable organization. Attendance at local chapter meetings is open, at no cost, to all individuals with an interest in the problem of impotence. Attendees have the option of placing their names on a chapter mailing list, which is kept strictly confidential.

Support groups, such as I.A., not only offer the opportunity for men and their partners to become better informed, but are also a unique outlet for individuals to share mutual problems. The following is the agenda of a fairly typical monthly meeting of the Atlanta, Georgia, I.A. chapter.

• Brief opening by the chapter coordinator

- VCR presentation of an educational film on impotence

- Lecture and slide presentation on impotence by a urologist

- Panel discussion — two couples relate their personal experiences

- Question-and-answer period, presided over by panel members and urologist

- Refreshments and informal discussion period

About 100 people attended this particular meeting, held in the cafeteria of a local hospital. Men made up slightly more than half the group. Most men were accompanied by their partners. The typical age of most present appeared to be in the thirty-five to fifty-five range, although many could have been considerably older or younger. About one out of ten in the group was black. From casual conversation during the discussion period, it was evident that individuals present were from virtually all walks of life, including business executives, teachers, professional athletes, entertainers, and construction workers.

Despite the sensitive nature of the subject, the attendees, as a whole, actively participated in the discussions. Questions asked at the meeting ranged from defining the reasonable expectations of sexual performance to the fine details involved in the selection and use of penile implants. Those present showed little hesitation to tackle two really sensitive issues — the cost of treatment, and what insurance companies will pay.

A typical meeting of Impotents Anonymous lasts about three hours. While there is never a charge for attendance, individuals can make a contribution to the refreshment fund. Meeting content varies, with the emphasis at many meetings on the psychological aspects of impotence.

Many attendees report that mere attendance at I.A.

meetings can offer a distinct feeling of relief, partly because of the realization that you are not alone in your problem. The atmosphere of good humor and fellowship prevailing at meetings is undoubtedly a factor, as is the feeling of relief at actually initiating action to solve an all-consuming problem.

Active attendance at Impotents Anonymous meetings is obviously not for everybody. The male and female lay coordinators of the Atlanta chapter have often provided useful information over the phone to both men and women who cannot or do not wish to attend meetings.

IMPOTENCE SUPPORT GROUPS
AND INFORMATION SOURCES

Organization/Address/ *Phone Number*	*Comments*
Impotents Anonymous (I.A.) 119 South Ruth Street Maryville, TN 37801 Phone: 615-983-6064	A support group established in 1981, with approximately 100 chapters. I-Anon is an affiliated organization for partners. A stamped, self-addressed envelope is suggested when requesting information.

Recovery of Male
    Potency (ROMP)
ROMP Center
Grace Hospital
18700 Meyers Road
Detroit, MI 48235
Phones: 800-835-7667
    313-966-3300
    (in Michigan)
	A support group established in 1983. ROMP currently is conducting self-help programs at twenty-three hospitals throughout the United States.

Organization/Address/ Phone Number	Comments
Potency Restored 8630 Fenton Street Suite 218 Silver Spring, MD 20910 Phone: 301-588-5777	A support group for couples established in 1981. The group meets monthly and offers a "total care program."
American Association of Sex Educators, Counselors and Therapists (AASECT) 11 Dupont Circle, N.W. Washington, DC 20036 Phone: 202-462-1171	The principal professional organization in the field. A national register is available of individuals meeting professional standards for membership.
American Urological Association 1120 North Charles St. Baltimore, MD 21201 Phone: 301-727-1100	The principal professional organization in the urology field. Information is also available from eight regional affiliates.
Impotence Information Center Department USA P.O. Box 9 Minneapolis, MN 55440 Phone: 800-843-4315	An information center provided by American Medical Systems, a leading manufacturer of penile prostheses.

This chapter has reviewed the basic options available to you if you seek help for a male sexual dysfunction problem. By learning as much as you can about your problem, asking the right questions (preferably in advance), and finding an informed physician, you can get the help you need.

CHAPTER 7

Treating impotence with hormones and drugs

For thousands of years, mankind has searched for a magical potion to cure impotence. Unfortunately, the results to date have been meager. At present, there are only a handful of hormones and drugs in the urologist's arsenal, of which testosterone, yohimbine, and papaverine are the most important. The pace of research is finally quickening, and it is expected that new and more effective drugs will become available over the next few years.

TESTOSTERONE

If you sample the blood testosterone levels of any large group of men of all ages and then plot, on a piece of graph paper, the level of testosterone versus age for each man, the result is a confused collection of dots scattered all over the piece of paper. Looking closer, or better still having a computer do the job for you, a pattern can be observed. Testosterone level is negligible below the age of ten. Then the level rises steeply through approximately age twenty-five. The rise continues, but at a much slower rate, to peak in the mid to late thirties. Then it declines slowly through the remaining years.

Confusion in the pattern occurs because many men differ widely from the norm. Occasionally, a man at age eighty may have double the testosterone level of most men of his age. On occasion, a man at age twenty-five may have half the normal level for his age. The wide variations are the result of a number of factors: disease, excessive use of alcohol, physical injury, or perhaps just the genes.

Phillip, a patient, age forty-two could not understand his lack of sexual drive, low level of energy, and lack of muscular strength. His blood testosterone level turned out to be only twenty-two, about the level of a ten-year-old boy. It should have been in excess of five hundred. Phillip was greatly helped by a testosterone supplementation program.

Before you conclude that testosterone is the cure for your problem, it is important to be aware of a few facts. Many men are able to perform very well despite abnormally low testosterone levels. Other men with abnormally low levels and sexual performance problems do not respond to the treatment. Testosterone supplementation does virtually nothing for men with normal levels. To make matters worse, excessive levels of testosterone supplementation can exacerbate prostatic cancer. Remember, castration is not uncommon in treating men for prostate cancer.

As a result, testosterone supplementation should be undertaken only under continuing medical direction. Unfortunately, it is sometimes possible to obtain the hormone without prescription.

There are basically three ways to replace deficient testosterone in the body. The first is to take the hormone orally. Oral tablets on the market are in the methyltestosterone form. Taking the drug orally is convenient, but it is not recommended, due to problems in controlling dosage levels. Some of the problems that may occur with improper usage include, in addition to the possibility of cancer, impaired liver function, and kidney damage.

A better way to raise your testosterone level is with intermuscular injections. This type of treatment starts with a series of trial injections in the urologist's office. The testosterone used is usually in the enanthate form. The dosage level initially used is in the 100 to 200 milligram range, depending upon your weight and the degree of deficiency. If the treatment is found to improve sexual performance, the injections are repeated every two weeks. Often, in addition to an improvement in performance, you may experience increased body vigor and a more enthusiastic mental state.

With suitable instructions, testosterone injections can continue at home, with the injections carried out either by you or by your partner. An alternative preferred by many patients is to have small, testosterone slow-release pellets implanted under the skin. The procedure is done in the urologist's office, takes about fifteen minutes and, except for the quick injection of a local anesthetic, is painless. The pellets are usually implanted in the upper back, a few inches below the left or right shoulder. Some patients experience swelling for a few days, itching, and minor discomfort. It is not a good time for weight lifting. Antibiotics are taken during this period to avoid infection. A testosterone pellet implant may prove effective for a period of six months to one year.

At the present time, experimental work is underway on the possible use of skin patches containing testosterone. If successful, this will permit the slow release of testosterone from a small adhesive patch placed on the scrotum.

Long-range work is currently underway in connection with the hormonal chemical known as LHRH. This chemical is believed to play a key role in the mechanism by which the pituitary gland, located in the base of the brain, controls the production of testosterone in the testicles. This work may ultimately result in a convenient way to raise hormonal levels.

YOHIMBINE

Yohimbine, usually in hydrochloride or lactate form, is a chemical substance that has some benefit in the treatment of impotence. This drug was originally obtained from the dried bark of the *corynanthe johimbe tree* found in various countries of central Africa. The drug can now be produced commercially by chemical synthesis.

For hundreds of years, yohimbine was used in folk medicine as an aphrodisiac. In fact, it was one of the few aphrodisiacs with any real evidence of effectiveness. Early in the twentieth century, the drug was used on a limited basis by physicians in the treatment of impotence. In the mid-1960s, the drug was rediscovered and used essentially on an experimental basis. Many of the recent studies have been based upon a drug with the brand name, Afrodex, a product that also contains methyltestosterone.

Yohimbine's aphrodisiac properties are believed to be due to the erotic effect the drug has on the brain and central nervous system. The drug's effectiveness in treating impotence, however, is believed to be related to its action in blocking the sympathetic nervous system, which in turn results in increased blood flow to the penis.

In general, yohimbine has been used most successfully in the treatment of impotent men with diabetes. The scientifically manufactured drug is available in tablet form from urologists. Ground johimbe tree bark, of questionable effectiveness, is sometimes available through health food stores and by mail order. Yohimbine must be used cautiously, and always under medical supervision. The drug has been found to increase blood pressure and, on occasion, cause nervousness. In fact, yohimbine has been used for the treatment of men and women with abnormally low blood pressure levels.

PAPAVERINE

Papaverine is a drug that acts as a vasodilator and muscle relaxant. It is used in the treatment of certain types of heart disease, and for arterial spasms occurring in the brain. It has been discovered in recent years that a solution of the drug injected directly in the corpora cavernosum region of the penis will initiate a firm and long-lasting erection. Investigation of this phenomenon has resulted in a workable treatment for impotence, a useful diagnostic tool, and a vast increase in the knowledge of the mechanics of erection that will pay off in future years.

Richard, a seventy-two-year-old patient, had been unable to achieve a firm erection for several years. After testing, his problem was found to be vascular or neurological in nature. Shortly after an injection of papaverine, Richard experienced an impressive erection that lasted for approximately three hours. After further testing and proper instructions, Richard was able to enjoy frequent and successful sexual activity at home.

An obvious problem in the use of papaverine is the perfectly understandable horror of most men at the thought of a penile injection. The fear, however, is far worse than the reality. Papaverine, sometimes in association with a second drug, Regitine (phentolamine), is injected into the side of the penis through a fine, small-gauge needle. The actual pain may be described as a slight pinch. After the first few times, almost all patients overcome their fear.

The use of papaverine involves the determination of proper dosage. After the first trial injection, the dosage level is experimentally increased or decreased until a level is obtained that results in an erection lasting about forty-five minutes. The patient is monitored very closely during the procedure, watching for the possibility of unwanted side effects.

Patients typically have little trouble in learning how to inject themselves at home in preparation for sexual activity. For home injection, one option is for the patient to obtain a supply of hypodermic syringes prefilled with the proper quantity of the drug. An alternative option is for the patient to fill empty syringes from a sterilized bottle containing a supply of the drug.

Although the use of penile injection may appear to be at odds with the fun and spontaneity of sexual relations, most men and their partners do not find this to be a deterrent. Many couples make a game of the procedure, turning it into an enjoyable experience.

Papaverine injection must always be used with caution, and all instructions should be carefully observed. An immediate problem can arise when an erection fails to relax over a prolonged period, such as up to six hours. This condition resembles priapism, but is normally not true priapism. Prolonged erections are rare, especially when instructions are followed.

Men who use injection therapy are instructed to contact their urologists promptly whenever an erection lasts more than four to six hours. Under such circumstances, the urologist usually terminates the erection with an injection of a diluted saline solution containing adrenalin (epinephrine). The injection neutralizes the effect of the papaverine, with the result that the dilated vessels carrying blood into the penis constrict, thus impeding the passage of blood into the penis. The urologist may also find it necessary to draw some blood out of the penis.

Using papaverine more than two times per week or at intervals of less than two days is not recommended, due to the possibility of scarring. Too-frequent use can also result in bruising, itching, and bleeding. Long-term use may result in fibrosis or scarring of the penis, or possibly a curved erection. The drug has also been found to gradually lose its effectiveness over a period of time.

In general, a papaverine injection provides a useful short-term solution for men who ultimately will elect to have a penile prosthesis installed, but wish to avoid immediate surgery. Although the drug has been approved by the U.S. Food and Drug Administration in connection with its traditional uses, penile injection therapy is still considered an experimental procedure that can be employed only under close medical supervision.

OTHER DRUGS

Several other drugs have been used for the treatment of impotence at least on an experimental basis. Bromocriptine mesylate, sold in tablets and capsules under the brand name Parlodel, for the treatment of female infertility and Parkinson's disease, has been found to improve erections in men with high levels of the female hormone prolactin. The drug lowers prolactin levels and improves erections even in men with pituitary tumors. Such tumors are associated with abnormal prolactin secretion into the bloodstream. When the underlying problem is a tumor, use of the drug does not substitute for direct treatment of the tumor itself.

Propylthiouracil is a drug used for the treatment of hyperthyroidism. This condition is sometimes linked to the loss of libido and erection difficulties. Use of the drug is often effective in improving both the thyroid and erection problem for many male patients.

Prostaglandin E_1 (alprostadil) is a drug normally used in the treatment of congenital heart defects in children. Some urologists recently have used the drug in penile injection therapy as a substitute for papaverine. Initial results have been encouraging. If experimental use demonstrates that postaglandin is safe and effective, it may someday be used in cases where papaverine does not provide a proper response or has lost its effectiveness after extended use.

Testosterone, yohimbine, and papaverine, the most important drugs being used today for impotence treatment, can yield good results in some patients. All three should be used with care and under a urologist's supervision. The newer, essentially experimental drugs also mentioned in this chapter should obviously be used with care and proper supervision. Nothing available to date is a universal cure-all, but help has been provided to many patients.

CHAPTER 8

Treating impotence surgically

*T*he following letter was received from a patient a few weeks after he had a penile implant:

Dear Doc,

I have to be careful not to sleep on my stomach anymore, inasmuch as I might puncture my water mattress.

You sure do good work, and now due to your good work, I'm doing pretty good work.

This chapter deals with the various surgical techniques now available for the treatment of impotence. Most of the chapter deals with prostheses that are surgically implanted in the penis. By definition, a prosthesis is any device that replaces or substitutes for a missing or nonworking body part. A dental plate is a common example of a prosthesis. A penile prosthesis is commonly referred to as a penile implant, or simply an implant.

Several surgical procedures being used to correct vascular problems linked to impotence are also discussed in this chapter. At present, there is little that can be done to deal surgically with neurological defects that result in impotence, although work on the repair of neurological damage, in general, is underway and is very promising.

The use of prostheses was pioneered in the United States, and has turned out to be the most common surgical solution to date for impotence among Americans. Vascular surgery for impotence was pioneered in Europe, and is most common with Europeans. In time, it is reasonable to expect that practice throughout the world will include the appropriate use of both approaches.

Finally, this chapter includes a brief discussion of external devices designed to provide an erection.

PENILE IMPLANTS

As noted in Chapter 2, penile implants have become available on a regular basis only since the 1970s. Since then, one estimate places the total number of devices that have been inserted in patients in the United States at about 150,000. The largest number of implants, about 29 percent, has been in the fifty to fifty-nine age group. Men age sixty to sixty-nine, account for about 23 percent, and the forty to forty-nine age group accounts for about 21 percent. Many men age seventy and older, however, have had implants, including quite a few men age eighty and older. Men with implants can father children. Recently this was the case with a twenty-nine-year-old patient who had never before been able to have successful sexual intercourse.

Several American companies are now manufacturing prostheses for a growing market. The rapid acceptance of implants reflects the fact that such devices represent a very pragmatic solution to the impotence problem. The single largest group of men who have chosen this solution is diabetics. Men who have undergone radical removal of the prostate, bladder, or colon represent the second largest group.

Types of implants

At present, three basic types of implants are available: the semirigid malleable prosthesis, the simple self-contained inflatable prosthesis, and the more complex three-piece inflatable prosthesis. Photographs of a product in each category, manufactured by American Medical Systems, Minneapolis, Minnesota, are shown on the following pages. The positioning of the inflatable implant within the penis and the lower body cavity is also shown in an accompanying drawing. A description of the types of implants and their respective advantages and disadvantages follows.

Semirigid malleable implant

Semirigid malleable implants, as shown in Figure 8-1, are relatively simple devices, and the first implants to be used on a large scale. Many different products of this nature have been developed by different manufacturers. Most semirigid implants supplied today are made of silicone, and incorporate a flexible metal core made of stainless steel or silver wire. Some are fabricated entirely from silicone, with no metal core.

When a semirigid malleable implant is surgically placed in the penis, a permanent erection results. The penis and implant can, however, be bent down close to the body so that it will not be noticed under most clothing. When intercourse is desired, the penis is merely straightened.

The principal advantage of a semirigid device is cost, both for the device itself and for implantation. The surgical procedure is simpler than with other types, and adapts to implantation on an outpatient basis. The principal disadvantage is the permanent erection. This could be a problem to a man when wearing a bathing suit or when changing clothes in a public locker room such as in a health club or gymnasium. The erection, while generally adequate,

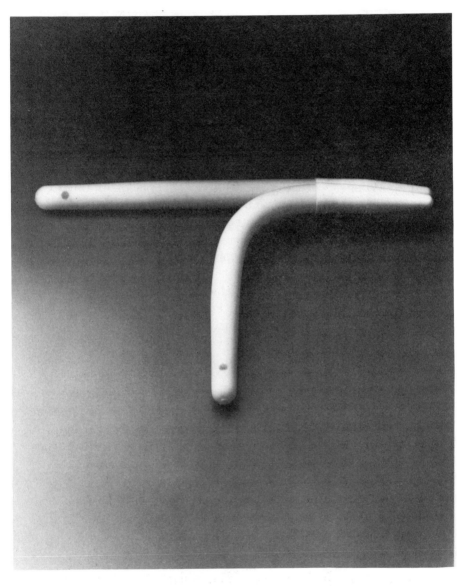

Figure 8-1
Semirigid Malleable Implant

Courtesy of American Medical Systems
Photograph by Mike Schenk

is not characterized by an increase in the length or girth of the penis. Finally, there is the remote possibility of perforation of the penis.

Simple self-contained inflatable implant

The simple self-contained inflatable implant, as shown in Figure 8-2, consists of two cylinders that are inserted entirely within the penis. Each cylinder contains hydraulic fluid. When an erection is desired, it is easily obtained by squeezing the end of each rod located near the front of the penis. The erection can be easily eliminated by bending the penis at its base, or by pressing the relief valves within the mechanism. The self-contained inflatable implant made its appearance in 1984.

The self-contained inflatable implant offers the advantage of an erection that can be controlled at will. As a consequence, there is no concealment problem. It is more expensive than the semirigid type, but less expensive than the more complex three-piece inflatable device. The surgical procedure required is relatively simple, although somewhat more complicated than with the semirigid malleable implant. A possible disadvantage is that it does not provide a particularly full erection, as there is no increase in the length or girth of the erect penis. However, this is rarely found to be a problem.

Three-piece inflatable implant

The three-piece inflatable implant, as shown in Figure 8-3, has been available since the mid-1970s. This device, which offers the best erection possible, contains three basic elements. The first element consists of two hollow cylinders that are placed within the penis. The second element is a pump and valve mechanism which is placed within the

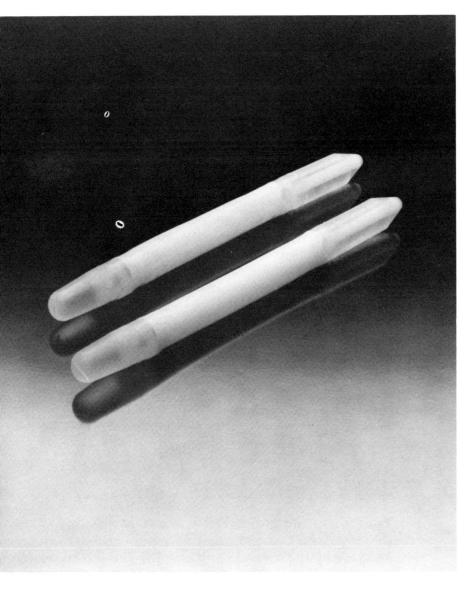

Figure 8-2
Simple, Self-Contained Inflatable Implant

Courtesy of American Medical Systems
Photograph by Mike Schenk

scrotum, close to the testicles. The third is a spherical reservoir containing hydraulic fluid, which is placed inside the lower abdomen. Three tubes, entirely inside the body, connect the reservoir to the pump and the pump to each cylinder. The hydraulic fluid used is a safe mixture of sterile water and diluted X-ray contrast material. The pump can be placed in either the right or left side of the scrotum, depending on personal preference.

This device is easily inflated by squeezing the pumping mechanism inside the scrotum, which results in fluid moving into the cylinders. When the erection is no longer desired, it is easily deactivated and the fluid returns to the reservoir.

The complex inflatable implant offers the advantages of maximum control and the most authentic-appearing erection. The resulting erection is characterized by both added penis length and increased girth. The disadvantages are higher cost and the more involved surgical procedure that is needed. Also, since the device is more complex, there is a greater possibility of malfunction. Despite these disadvantages, however, the majority of men are choosing the complex inflatable implant.

Continuing product improvement, including design changes and the use of superior materials, has resulted in less time needed in surgery and greatly reduced occurrence of malfunction. Simpler two-piece devices have also become available.

Implant surgery

Both the semirigid and the simple self-contained inflatable prostheses are inserted surgically through an opening made by the surgeon in the penis. The procedure is relatively simple.

The implantation of an inflatable prothesis of the non-self-contained type is the most complicated procedure, and is usually performed in a hospital setting. A skilled urologist,

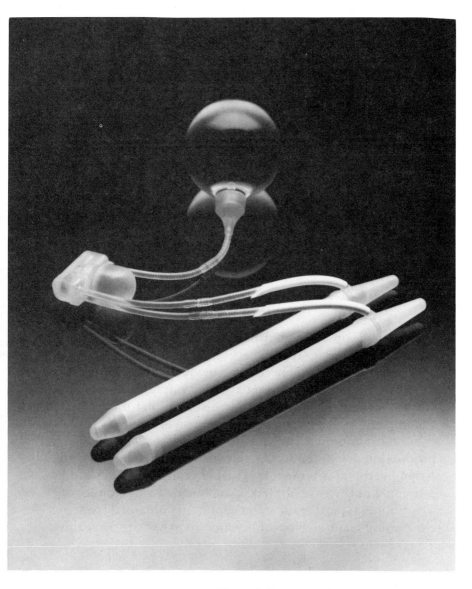

Figure 8-3
Three-Piece Inflatable Implant

Courtesy of American Medical Systems
Photograph by Mike Schenk

however, can perform the procedure in as little as thirty minutes and, in many instances, on an outpatient basis. Depending on the preferred procedure, the device is inserted through a small opening below the base of the penis or in the lower abdominal cavity. The three major elements of the device are then placed in the desired positions, as shown in Figure 8-4.

In the surgical procedure, the patient does not have to have general anesthesia, as the use of a spinal or local type of anesthesia is possible. Some patients, of course, may prefer full anesthesia. Patients typically are hospitalized for one to three days. Most patients are back to work in one week. Full recovery may take up to four weeks, and sexual intercourse should be possible by the fourth to sixth week. Patients receive careful instructions for the recovery period.

The results

Based on information provided by the author's patients, favorable results are reported in excess of 90 percent of the cases. There is no evidence that the implant interferes with normal sexual intercourse. Patients who were able to achieve orgasm or ejaculate before receiving the implant are fully capable of doing so afterwards.

As mentioned previously, men with adequate sperm production are perfectly capable of fathering children after having received an implant. This, of course, obviously does not apply in the case of men who have had vasectomies.

Some typical results and comments obtained from our continuing mail survey of former patients are revealing. These include:

Question: *Are you satisfied with how hard your penis is when it is in the "up" position?*

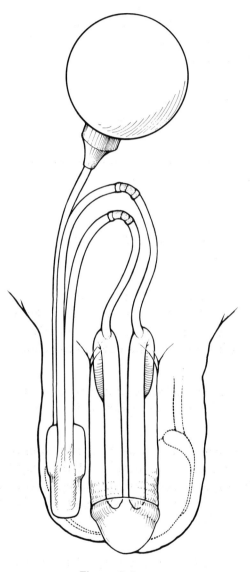

Figure 8-4
Drawing Showing Location of Inflatable
Implant Within the Body

Courtesy of American Medical Systems
Photograph by Mike Schenk

Almost all former patients check the "yes" answer. A patient who qualified a positive response with the word "almost," nevertheless indicated strong general satisfaction in subsequent questions.

> Question: *Are you satisfied with how your penis looks*
>   *in the "down" position?*

The answers to this question are almost unanimously positive. Comments range from "very" to "it is A-okay" to "mighty proud."

> Question: *Overall, are you happier since your penile*
>   *implant?*

Again the response is almost always "yes." Some comments include "much," "very," and "definitely." One especially articulate former patient commented as follows: "Absolutely. It's like getting the keys to the candy store."

> Question: *Knowing what you know now, would you*
>   *still have decided to have an implant?*

The response to this question is strongly positive. Comments range from a simple "damn right" to the following: "I'm only sorry I did not know of this technique sooner! I feel and believe I act younger . . . All impotent men should have this!"

> Question: *If such a thing were possible, is there*
>   *anything you would change about your*
>   *prosthesis?*

Almost all responses to this final question were

negative. An articulate patient added the comments, "I am completely happy with it, and so is my wife. I don't know how it could be improved." According to another patient: "It's the only operation I've ever enjoyed." A third patient: "I should have had it done ten years ago."

The implant decision

The decision to have an implant should never be taken lightly. It is a decision that involves a major medical procedure and financial expense, as well as the patient's partner and life style. Any man considering an implant should be well informed on the subject, and review all aspects of the matter with his urologist and his partner. Talking to men who have had implants, and their partners, can also be very useful. Such people can be contacted through impotence support groups. Some factors that will influence the implant decision are illustrated by the following examples.

CASE 1 — A MAN WITH NO OTHER CHOICE

Larry, a sixty-year-old truck driver, very much desired to have sexual relations with his partner, but this had not been possible for the past five years. Unfortunately, his impotence was due to irreversible physical damage resulting from alcoholism. Fortunately, he had stopped drinking. It was too late however, for Larry ever again to enjoy normal sexual activity, unless he were to receive an implant.

CASE 2 — A MAN WITH LIMITED CHOICE

Walter, a retired sixty-eight-year-old corporate executive, had been experiencing impotence for about two years. He was in excellent health, and medical examinations revealed no physical condition that could be connected to impotence. A good possibility existed that Walter's problem was psychological in nature, possibly associated with life-style changes necessitated by retirement.

Walter chose an implant over some form of psychological or sex therapy. A very private and strong-minded person, Walter objected to any form of treatment that would involve the exposure of his feelings. He reasoned, probably correctly, that given his general attitudes, he would be a very poor candidate for successful treatment of a psychological nature. In Walter's words, "At my age, anything other than an implant would be a waste of time and money."

CASE 3 — A MAN WITH A POSSIBLY VIABLE ALTERNATIVE

Charles, a thirty-five-year-old university professor, had been experiencing impotence symptoms for about six months. When examined, he was in generally good health, although he had been drinking and smoking more than usual since the impotence problem began. No definite physical problem linked to impotence could be detected by examination.

Charles was anxious to have an implant. He was encouraged, however, to first undertake a program of sex therapy and to defer a possible implant until the results of such treatment became apparent. The results were favorable and an implant was not found to be necessary.

Some common concerns about penile implants

Concern 1 — I would like an implant, but I am, frankly, worried about the operation. Is it safe? What will happen? Will it be painful? Will anybody find out?

All surgical procedures have some degree of risk. Even

in a very simple operation, such as having your tonsils taken out, occasionally a patient will have an adverse reaction to the anesthesia. Local infection is a possibility, and does occur in roughly 1 percent to 2 percent of the cases. In such cases, it may be necessary to repeat the surgical procedure at a later time.

The most involved of the procedures requires being admitted to the hospital as an inpatient. In this case, the patient is admitted to the hospital on the morning of the surgery or perhaps the night before. Routine tests and a preoperative examination are performed. The patient will be visited by an anesthesiologist, and anesthesia options will be fully discussed. Usually, the patient will receive one or more injections of intravenous antibiotics prior to the operation and, when desired, an injection of a suitable tranquilizer.

The operation itself is not especially painful, as it is done with appropriate anesthesia. The patient is usually on his feet and getting around easily shortly after the operation. The patient is also usually able to resume eating on the day of surgery. Some mild localized discomfort is common during the recovery period, associated with the healing incision. The pain and discomfort gradually diminish and, in any event, can be controlled with suitable medication. When healing is complete and pain fully disappears, the patient is no longer aware of the presence of the implant. The situation is much the same as wearing a wristwatch — it is something that you are not aware of until you want to use it.

Privacy is a very real and justifiable concern of most men. The time spent in the hospital, and the overall recovery period, are sufficiently short so that the entire matter can take place during a brief vacation period. This was Donald's approach. The fifty-year-old business executive checked into the hospital over the Christmas holidays. He commented that he was giving a Christmas present to himself. The only people who ever knew he was there were the involved medical personnel, the insurance company, and his partner.

Concern 2 — Will my partner find the implant somehow objectionable?

No statistical survey of partners has ever been conducted which would answer this question conclusively. There is, however, considerable case evidence, based on interviews with partners and comments made at meetings of impotence support groups, that the entire sexual process feels natural and fully satisfactory. Some female partners comment that with the implant the pressure to perform is removed, allowing both partners to find the sexual experience more enjoyable than ever before.

Actually, there is very little obvious evidence of the existence of an implant. In rare instances, some men with implants have reported that partners who have not been made aware of the existence of the implant have not suspected its presence.

Concern 3 — Is it "natural"?

Walter, a patient with vascular insufficiency, was worried that a penile implant is "just not natural." Walter explained that he would only buy "natural" vitamins and other products at a health food store. He would wear only clothes made of wool and cotton, never synthetics. He proudly advised that he would never use pesticides or synthetic fertilizers on the tomato plants he grew each year. Walter, however, also wore glasses, had several dental crowns, and had been inoculated against all the common contagious diseases.

A penile implant, of course, is not natural, in much the same sense that riding in an automobile or flying in an airplane is not natural. It does, however, allow a man to engage in normal sexual activity that feels natural in all respects. Walter's actual problem was that he had been conditioned to believe that a *real* man never has trouble achieving a supererection. It never occurred to Walter that if sex is only to be performed under perfectly natural conditions, all forms of contraception would be automatically ruled out, including abstinence from sex during the female partner's fertile periods. After a successful implant, Walter was the first to admit he had been wrong.

Concern 4 — I am a very active person. Will the presence of an implant cause a problem?

Men with implants include heavy construction workers and at least one professional wrestler, and they normally have no difficulty in engaging in vigorous sports, including running, tennis, weight lifting, and bicycle riding. There is, of course, the "locker room problem" associated with the semirigid prosthesis, as discussed previously.

Few sports place as much physical stress on the groin area as horseback riding and polo do. Yet one former implant patient continues to play a vigorous game of polo, and reports no unfavorable consequences.

Concern 5 — I feel guilty about the expense.

Money is always a consideration. As seen in Chapter 11, the total expense after insurance is not unreasonable. The enjoyment of normal sexual activity is not a personal indulgence, but an essential part of life for most adults in our society. The cost of treatment is actually less than the emotional cost of nontreatment.

Concern 6 — I feel guilty about not solving the emotional problems causing my condition.

This statement implies a belief that impotence is always caused by psychological factors. This, as you now know, is definitely not the case. Some sex therapists will hint that it is a sign of weakness to decide on an implant, rather than embark on a program of sex therapy, when the underlying problem appears to be entirely psychological. In the case of older men, with obviously limited life expectancy, the choice of an implant can be very logical and certainly nothing to feel guilty about.

Concern 7 — Will problems develop using the implant?

The chemically inert materials used in available prostheses, especially silicone, have been carefully selected to avoid health hazards. Similar materials are regularly placed inside the body in connection with other forms of medical treatment, without problems developing.

There is, as previously discussed, a possibility of the implanted prosthesis malfunctioning, which will necessitate surgical removal and replacement. This, as noted, is becoming far less common, due to continuing improvements in technology.

Some patients feel that the possibility of a malfunctioning prosthesis is a small price to pay for regained sexual vigor. For example, Bernie had been very pleased with his implant, but, to his considerable regret, the device stopped working after five months. X-ray examination revealed that there was a rupture in the cylinder, and the hydraulic fluid had escaped. Without hesitation, Bernie decided on a prompt replacement, which has provided excellent service for the past three years. Bernie views the matter philosophically, advising that he has twice replaced defective fuel pumps in an expensive late-model automobile.

A second problem is that a relatively small number of men have difficulty adjusting to the idea that an implanted device is substituting for what they think should be a natural consequence of their manhood. At times, such men become morbidly preoccupied with the presence of the implant. This problem can only be avoided if the urologist carefully screens patients before the operation. In many instances, this type of problem is due to unrealistic expectations as to how the implant will change the man's life.

VASCULAR SURGERY

Vascular surgery for impotence falls into two categories: procedures involving the venous system (which drains blood out of the penis), and procedures involving the arterial system (which supplies blood to the penis). Both approaches are very promising, although there is a considerable amount of work that has to be done before vascular surgery, in general, becomes a major solution for the impotence problem. Most work in the field has taken place only during the past ten years.

Much of what is known regarding surgical procedures to correct abnormal drainage of blood from the penis has been learned as a result of treatment to correct the consequences of priapism. In treating an emergency priapism episode, the temporary drainage channel made by the physician to draw off blood may fail to heal properly, and persistent blood leakage and impotence may be the unfortunate result. The procedure to treat this condition is not difficult, and can be performed under local anesthesia. In the operation, the surgeon makes an incision near the front of the penis, and cuts through to the damaged area that has been previously located by a corpora cavernosagram. The open channel is then sutured, resulting in the elimination of the leak.

The problem becomes more complicated when the patient has not experienced priapism, but a drainage problem is evident. The problem in these cases is accurately pinpointing the open channel or channels responsible for the problem. When the area of leakage can be properly identified from a corpora cavernosagram, the repair is usually successful.

This was the case with Wayne, age sixty-five, who had originally been scheduled for a penile implant. A second opinion revealed a simple leakage problem. A successful repair was achieved with a fifteen-minute surgical procedure.

Surgery to correct most arterial problems represents a major medical procedure, and is still at an early stage of development. One approach has been attempting to bypass the area where the critical arteries are blocked or are too narrow to permit adequate flow of blood to the penis. The bypass approach would be potentially most useful in treating impotence caused by arteriosclerosis. Unfortunately, this approach has not proven highly successful, although there is long-range promise as surgical techniques improve.

Greater success has been achieved in the surgical removal of lesions impeding blood flow. Such lesions are usually caused by physical injury, and represent a frequent cause of impotence in younger men.

EXTERNAL DEVICES

External devices that may be placed around the penis in order to sustain an erection are sometimes advertised in questionable publications. Such devices are usually ineffective. In the case of so-called "cock" rings, they can be dangerous. For example, after Roger appeared in the office with three permanent bends in his penis, it took an involved surgical procedure to literally straighten him out. Eventually, Roger had to have an implant to properly restore sexual function.

There are, however, several legitimate products that have been developed. One such device resembles a condom, and is placed over the penis. The device serves to constrict the penis, which results in a buildup of pressure at the base of the penis. The device incorporates a tube that permits the use of suction to draw blood into the penis. The blood is entrapped due to the pressure at the base of the penis.

Vacuum and entrapment devices are not widely used. They do, however, offer an option for some men.

At present, the penile implant represents the most workable solution for an impotence problem for most patients. Patients have available several good choices as to type of implant. An overwhelming number of patients report satisfaction after having received an implant. Problems associated with implants are relatively infrequent.

Surgical approaches to the treatment of impotence, involving vascular surgery, are still at an early stage of development. In time, such approaches can be expected to yield useful alternatives to penile implants in some patients.

CHAPTER 9

Treating impotence with psychotherapy and sex therapy

This chapter describes the principal methods currently being used for the treatment of impotence presumably of a psychological origin. These treatments include traditional psychotherapy and more contemporary treatment methods commonly grouped under the term "sex therapy."

It should again be emphasized that no extensive treatment program for impotence that involves psychoanalysis or some form of sex therapy should be undertaken until the possibility of an identifiable physical cause is completely ruled out. Failure to do so could result in a delay in obtaining effective treatment, unnecessary emotional stress, and considerable expense. Any responsible psychotherapist or sex therapist will make this point clear to all prospective patients. However, if the condition is causing relationship problems, psychoanalysis can be very helpful.

In general, the number of accurate scientific studies of the effectiveness of psychological treatments for impotence has been limited. The studies that are available often reveal a mixed pattern of success. The chances for success are logically best in the case of men with impotence of a psychological origin and no evidence of any physical problem causing the impotence. It is also logical that some men with psychological impotence and only borderline physical problems may be helped to some extent.

USE OF TRADITIONAL PSYCHOTHERAPY

As observed in Chapter 2, traditional psychoanalytical theory originally attributed impotence to the existence of unconscious conflict arising from the incest taboo and various traumatic childhood sexual experiences. In time, the explanation was broadened to include other possible causes, such as repressed anger against a partner and general feelings of incompetence. The psychoanalytic process is intended to uncover these underlying experiences, and with this knowledge it is anticipated that the impotence problem will disappear.

The basic format employed in traditional one-on-one psychotherapy is familiar to most persons and need not be discussed here in depth. A man subject to impotence problems who elects such therapy can usually look forward to several preliminary forty-five to fifty minute sessions with the therapist, devoted to taking a detailed personal history and to reviewing past and present physical and emotional problems. In subsequent sessions, the patient is encouraged to freely discuss, in an essentially unstructured manner, memories of past events, relationships with others, personal fears, dreams, current conscious experiences, and so forth.

Therapy sessions continue on this basis indefinitely. In highly traditional therapy, sessions may occur at the rate of as many as four sessions per week. With other therapists, the sessions may be scheduled at the rate of one per week.

There is usually some time off during the course of the year to allow for the therapist's vacation periods.

Some therapists suggest that a period of at least two years is required before any tangible progress can be experienced, arguing that it takes at least that long for the patient to overcome inhibitions and freely confide to his therapist his most intimate personal feelings. According to traditional psychoanalytical theory, the patient gradually develops a strong dependence on the therapist during the course of the sessions. With the subsequent achievement of insight, the patient finds himself relieved of a wide spectrum of psychological problems, including impotence. In time, the patient is also able to function without the support of the therapist, and therefore will be eventually in a position to discontinue treatment. The entire process may take years.

The interpretation of dreams has been a key element in traditional psychotherapy. This is based on the belief that dreams provide access to important, but threatening, matters that are repressed by the conscious mind. Patients are encouraged to write down dream sequences promptly upon awakening, for later discussion at therapy sessions. Various symbolic images appearing in dreams are believed to be representative of important psychological factors, and are therefore of great significance in dream interpretation.

Current research on artificial intelligence systems, as employed in the computer field, suggests interesting insights into the functioning of the intelligence system of the human brain. This research raises some doubt as to the general area of dream interpretation. Artificial intelligence systems have a finite capacity, and thus are prone to disruption when computer electronic memory circuits are overloaded with information. The memory circuits of the human brain are also finite. Dreams could merely be a routine mechanism for the purging of extraneous information to make room for new information. Should this theory prove valid, it could follow that dreams hardly provide a window on the human mind. In fact, dreams might be somewhat analogous to the confused jumble of characters sometimes seen on computer displays, known to computer hackers as "garbage."

Can psychotherapy in practice actually help men with psychological impotence? The answer appears to be yes, although the process may prove tortuous. In one report that appeared in medical literature in 1972, about one-fourth of a study group of men with impotence problems experienced some improvement after being in therapy at the rate of four sessions per week over a period of at least two years. Improvement was also experienced in about one-half of a group who had received less intensive therapy.

Given the high degree of personal commitment that is implied in undertaking any extensive program of psychotherapy, men with true psychological impotence are well advised to carefully consider their overall situation. Psychotherapy is designed to simultaneously treat a wide variety of problems. Under these circumstances, the use of psychotherapy for the treatment of impotence alone can prove unsuccessful on a cost-effective basis. On the other hand, a man with psychological impotence plus a wide variety of other emotional problems that are sufficiently serious to justify treatment, might conclude that the overall benefits would make a program of psychotherapy worthwhile.

SENSATE FOCUS THERAPY

Variations exist in the treatment programs employing the sensate focus approach made popular by Masters and Johnson. Typically, such programs are short, but intensive in nature, and involve lengthy interactive discussions with sex therapists, education in sexual matters, and graduated sexual exercises. The educational component is intended to overcome misconceptions about sex, which are believed to contribute in some manner to inadequate sexual perform-ance. The exercise component is designed to overcome the problem of performance anxiety. Most sensate focus therapy programs involve the active participation of male and female partners, usually a married couple, throughout the treatment process.

As discussed in Chapter 3, sensate focus therapy is largely a result of Masters and Johnson studies conducted during the 1960s. Most current sensate focus treatment programs today are heavily influenced by the original Masters and Johnson treatment model. The treatment was designed to deal with the sexual problems of both men and women and a variety of dysfunction problems. The original Masters and Johnson treatment model consisted of fourteen consecutive days of intensive therapy for both partners. Participants were encouraged to regard the experience as a vacation or retreat free from such day-to-day distractions as children and employment. Such conditions were believed to maximize the possibility of treatment success.

Couples participating in the program spent their first three days providing medical histories, undergoing physical examinations, and participating in intensive discussions with an assigned male and female co-therapy team. By the third day, they were instructed to begin simple and nondemanding sexual exercises, but with all genital contact discouraged. On the fourth day, the participants received specific instructions for the remainder of the program, tailored toward the particular problem to be overcome (impotence, premature ejaculation, and so forth). The remaining days of the program were largely devoted to sexual exercises conducted in private by the participating couple, but with the availability of the co-therapist team for active consultation and advice.

The key element in the general Masters and Johnson approach, as it is employed today, is the gradual and nondemanding nature of the prescribed sexual exercises. Initial exercises are typically limited to the simple stroking of nongenital body parts, such as the face and back. Genital contact, when finally established, proceeds from mild touching. The female partner is instructed to carefully avoid the verbal and nonverbal communication of personal sexual demands. When attempted intercourse seems propitious, the position with the female astride the male is prescribed, in order to minimize stress on the male. Use of other positions and attendance to the female's needs is suggested only during the advanced stages of the treatment program.

Brief mention should be made regarding the use of female surrogates, which has been sensationalized in the media. Use of such surrogates, at least by Masters and Johnson, has been largely limited to men subject to primary impotence. Such men, given their problem, often do not have an ongoing relationship with a female partner. Presumably, there is no effective way to help such men without provision for a surrogate. The use of surrogates obviously should be avoided unless the surrogate is very well-trained and subject to the supervision of a qualified sex therapist.

Variations of the sensate focus approach involve departures from the original fourteen-day format, supplementing the treatment program with various elements derived from traditional psychotherapy, behavioral therapy, biofeedback, and hypnosis. Dr. Bernie Zilbergeld, a California-based sex therapist, has suggested a series of sexual exercises that emphasize the use of masturbation. Some of Zilbergeld's exercises in this co-author's opinion, appear to be bizarre. For example, in one suggested exercise, the patient is asked to compose a letter from the penis to its owner, expressing a series of grievances.

How effective is sensate focus therapy? The original Masters and Johnson studies reported a success rate in the treatment of impotence in the range of approximately 60 percent to 70 percent. Stated another way, this implies failure in about one-third of the patients. The criteria for measuring success in the studies was fairly modest, being the ability to maintain an erection throughout intercourse at least 25 percent of the time. From a cost-benefit standpoint, successful sensate focus therapy appears to offer an advantage over traditional psychotherapy in the specific treatment of psychological impotence. Of course, it does not provide, as a byproduct, the treatment of other problems of an emotional nature.

OTHER TREATMENTS

Various other treatments of a psychological nature have been attempted for impotence. One such approach is behavior therapy, which employs systematic conditioning techniques, with the intention of modifying some undesired aspect of human behavior. In the motion picture *A Clockwork Orange*, the general public was exposed to a provocative example of the use of behavior therapy in the treatment of antisocial behavior.

The treatment of impotence with behavior therapy generally revolves around some scheme to overcome performance anxiety. In a typical approach, the patient is first encouraged to completely relax. Sometimes appropriate drugs are used to assist relaxation. The patient is then asked to imagine or actually view a series of sexual images. The images are arranged in order of increasing sexual explicitness, and are therefore intended to present increasing anxiety to the patient. No new image, however, is presented until the patient is able to cope with the previous image without anxiety.

The theory is that the patient, when ultimately desensitized to the most erotic and threatening sexual image in the series, will be able to perform with a partner in an actual sexual situation. One study has reported some degree of improvement in about three-quarters of a group of men treated for impotence in this manner.

Biofeedback is a fairly recent concept that involves training individuals to control various bodily functions which are capable of being monitored in some manner. Biofeedback, for example, has been used with some degree of success in the treatment of hypertension. In this particular case, patients are trained in appropriate techniques to control their blood pressure levels, with continuous measurements of blood pressure providing an immediate indication of the degree of success in achieving control.

The use of biofeedback in the treatment of impotence has typically involved the imagining or actual viewing of erotic sexual images, accompanied by the continuous monitoring of penile physical dimensions to indicate erectile success. If the treatment proves successful, the patient, over a period of time, is expected to gradually achieve some degree of control over the ability to achieve an erection, and is able to carry over this control into an actual sexual situation. Studies to date of the use of biofeedback training in the treatment of impotence are inconclusive, but generally discouraging.

Hypnotherapy has sometimes been attempted in the treatment of impotence. Hypnotism is an old technique that has been used on occasion for legitimate medical purposes. On the other hand, hypnotism has all too often been the province of the quack or stage performer.

Hypnotherapy has sometimes been used in the treatment of psychological impotence, in combination with traditional psychotherapy. The inducement of a hypnotic state has been used to identify deeply repressed experiences that may underlie the impotence problem. Attempts have also been made to induce erections in patients under hypnosis. Individual cases have been reported of successful treatment of impotence using hypnotherapy. However, conclusive scientific evidence demonstrating the positive value of hypnotherapy is lacking to date.

In general, behavior therapy, biofeedback training, and hypnotherapy should be approached with caution. Behavior therapy and biofeedback training should be regarded as essentially experimental techniques at this time. While hypnotherapy has existed for some time, the lack of serious ongoing scientific research in this field is grounds for concern. Men with impotence problems are advised to steer clear of such treatments, unless offered under the auspices of a highly regarded medical center and by practitioners with verifiable credentials.

CHAPTER 10

Treating other male sexual dysfunction problems

lthough this book deals primarily with the impotence problem, other forms of male sexual dysfunction can be as troubling to both the afflicted man and his partner. In many cases, such problems may lead to impotence of either a physical or psychological nature.

TREATING PREMATURE EJACULATION

After impotence, premature ejaculation is the male sexual dysfunction that receives the most attention. When premature ejaculation episodes multiply, especially in older men never previously subject to the problem, it makes sense to check for a possible prostate infection.

Prostate infections can be quite difficult to detect. In fact, a man can harbor a low grade infection without knowing it. Such men may feel generally run-down, but may exhibit little in the way of overt symptoms. Actually, premature ejaculation may be the only symptom. As a consequence, it is a good idea, especially for older men, to have frequent prostate examinations to detect possible infection or a more serious problem.

A full examination requires the physician to probe the gland through the anus, and also to exert pressure, with massage, to force a small quantity of fluid through the penis. The fluid is then examined in the laboratory to make a definitive determination of infection. As the process is unpleasant to many men, ultrasonic devices are being developed to permit noninvasive scanning of the prostate. Ultrasonic scanning, while potentially useful, will not substitute for the fluid-collecting process.

One reason why the prostate is subject to infection is that its internal structure allows disease-causing microorganisms to collect. There is, unfortunately, not much that can be done at this time to prevent infections of this nature from occurring. Frequent massage of the prostate gland encourages drainage, but it is obviously impractical.

Most prostate infections are easily cured by antibiotics. During treatment, the prescribed drug must be taken for the full amount of time specified, and alcohol should be avoided, as it often interferes with the action of many antibiotics. Treatment requires follow-up prostate examination, to make sure the infection has been fully eliminated.

After treatment, premature ejaculation should disappear, assuming the infection was the real cause of the problem. As a byproduct, after treatment many men feel much healthier, as they have eliminated something that had been adversely affecting their overall system. Curing a prostate infection, however, may have no effect on an impotence problem.

If a physical problem does not exist, sex therapy or more psychotherapy can be tried. In sex therapy, a variety of approaches are used, depending upon the therapist, including masturbation exercises. The Masters and Johnson approach for the treatment of premature ejaculation, in its early stages, is identical to the one used for treating impotence (see Chapter 9). At some point in the treatment, the female partner is directed to assume a "training" position. In this position, the woman is seated with her legs apart and her back pressed against the headboard of the bed. Her partner lies on his back with his pelvic area facing upward between her legs. In this position, she has easy access to her partner's penis and can conveniently employ a penile "squeeze" technique designed to retard ejaculation.

Unfortunately, the squeeze and other techniques often do not work. In such cases, penile injection therapy using the drug papaverine may be helpful. With the injection and subsequent extended erection, the patient with a psychological premature ejaculation problem is able to achieve vaginal penetration regardless of when ejaculation actually occurs. Success of this nature raises the patient's confidence, and the problem may eventually disappear.

A variety of quack remedies for premature ejaculation, such as numbing creams, are available. These remedies are by and large useless — some potentially dangerous — and they should be avoided.

TREATING RETROGRADE EJACULATION

Retrograde ejaculation presumably could be treated with surgery to strengthen the defective sphincter muscle that is allowing seminal fluid to pass into the bladder. There has been little incentive to develop this surgical technique, as retrograde ejaculation does not represent a threat to health, and an alternative exists for dealing with the problem faced by men who wish to have children.

Fortunately, most men who suffer from retrograde ejaculation following prostate surgery are of the age where children are no longer desired. When the problem results from a physical injury, it is more likely that the victim is a younger man desiring children. In such cases, the ability to father children can be achieved by collecting the first passage of urine from the bladder following ejaculation. The sperm can then be filtered out of the urine in the laboratory and used to artificially inseminate the female partner. Although the esthetics can be troubling to some persons, the approach is effective as long as there is no defect with the sperm. As to any doubt that sperm can survive the brief period of immersion in urine, consider the ability of sperm to overcome chemical and physical barriers presented in many forms of birth control.

There is a possibility that the lack of visible ejaculate may trouble some men, or even their partners. This could be the case with a man who feels compelled to feign orgasm, out of a mistaken belief that its absence somehow indicates personal failure. This is a problem to be solved by greater communication between the partners, and possibly by counseling.

TREATING EJACULATORY FAILURE

Treatment of the anorgasmic male has not received the attention that it deserves, due to the fairly rare occurrence of persistent ejaculatory failure. This is unfortunate, as effective treatment can be difficult to accomplish while, at the same time, the condition is very troubling to afflicted men and their partners.

In treating failure to ejaculate, it is logical to first check for any possible hormonal or neurological abnormality, and to treat any condition uncovered whenever possible. There is little difficulty in identifying the cause of the problem when there has been a recent major spinal injury. When there is nerve damage from an old forgotten injury of childhood, identification is more difficult.

As a result of continuing research in rehabilitation medicine, it is no longer hopeless when a man with a spinal injury and his partner want children. A technique now exists in which electrodes are implanted in critical nerve areas controlling ejaculation. When a small electrical charge is applied, ejaculation results.

The ejaculate is then collected and used to artificially inseminate the female partner. Electroejaculation will not result in the pleasurable sensations of orgasm, but the ability to have children will greatly enrich the lives of couples faced with these unfortunate circumstances. It is most likely that research in the general area will ultimately lead to workable treatment methods for all anorgasmic men.

When a physical cause cannot be identified, and the problem is presumed to be psychological in nature, sex therapy may prove useful. Masters and Johnson report a high degree of success in the treatment of the problem. The Masters and Johnson treatment for ejaculatory failure, as in the case for premature ejaculation, follows the same general format, in the beginning, as in the treatment of impotence. At an intermediate point in the program, the male partner is encouraged to masturbate to ejaculation in the presence of his partner. Subsequently, the female partner is expected to manipulate the penis to a point approaching ejaculatory inevitability, and rapidly mount the male and position the penis in her vagina just prior to ejaculation. The initial manipulation of the penis and the pelvic thrusting after vaginal penetration by the female should be performed in a "demanding" manner. With patience and repeated practice, this approach is expected to result in an eventual resolution of the problem.

TREATING PRIAPISM

Priapism is always an emergency medical procedure. As a result, men at higher risk, such as victims of sickle-cell anemia, are well advised to be aware of the possibility. It is also important for such men to insist upon treatment by a urologist when seeking treatment in a hospital emergency room.

The treatment of priapism is essentially the same as that described in Chapter 7 in connection with the treatment of a prolonged erection that may occur in penile injection therapy. It includes the injection of adrenalin (epinephrine), and possibly drawing blood from the penis. The prospects for successful treatment are obviously much greater for men with a prolonged erection after a penile injection, as such men are under the continuing care of a urologist, know what to expect, and have rapid access to a specialist in an emergency.

TREATING PEYRONIE'S DISEASE

The scarring of the penis characteristic of Peyronie's disease will often disappear on its own, in time, leaving no lasting problems. For this reason, when the visible symptoms are first noted and do not cause a problem, a urologist may suggest carefully observing the situation for a reasonable period of time.

If treatment is necessary, the most effective current approach is surgery. Most surgical procedures involve the removal of the plaque and the grafting of skin over the affected area. A penile implant may be required when there is a simultaneous impotence problem.

Several other treatments that have been tried unfortunately are often ineffective. These include the use of steroid injections, ultrasound, and vitamin E therapy. Treatment with potassium aminobenzoate, a drug sold under the brand name Potaba, has sometimes proven effective. The drug, which is available in tablets, is most often used in the treatment of various dermatological diseases. Experimental work is underway on treatments that involve the injection of certain enzymes known to dissolve scar tissues.

TREATING PAINFUL EJACULATION

Usually, painful ejaculation is easily treated with antibiotics when the problem is due to a prostate infection.

(Treatment of prostate infections is described in connection with premature ejaculation.)

If no physical cause can be found, it may be assumed that the problem is psychological. If the problem persists over an extended period, psychotherapy may be indicated.

Painful ejaculation and blood in the urine, also a symptom of prostate infection, should always be medically investigated. The reason is not only the possible long-range consequences of prostate infection, but also the very real possibility that these problems could result in loss of desire, performance anxiety, and even psychological impotence.

TREATING LACK OF DESIRE

Lack of desire obviously is a psychological problem, but one that can very well have a physical cause. It is therefore advisable to first determine whether a physical problem exists. When there are hormonal abnormalities, such as elevated prolactin or depressed testosterone levels, the problem may disappear with appropriate hormonal therapy. When lack of desire is the psychological response to impotence caused by physical factors, the logical approach is the appropriate treatment of the impotence problem. If lack of desire is associated with depression, it is advisable to promptly investigate the depression in its own right.

Simple family counseling may be helpful when there is reason to believe the problem is purely psychological and results from some failure in a stable and mutually desired relationship between two partners. If the problem is more deep-seated, appropriate psychotherapy may be required, especially when there is depression for which there is no apparent physical explanation.

TREATING PERFORMANCE ANXIETY

Performance anxiety is another example of a psychological problem that can often have a physical cause. Treating the physical problem often overcomes the performance anxiety. For example, Norman, age fifty-five, became increasingly anxious after repeated episodes of premature ejaculation. He feared the possible ridicule of his much younger wife. Eventually he avoided all sexual activity. Norman's problem was due to a prostate infection. When this was cured, his fears as to proper performance were overcome, and normal sexual activities were resumed.

When it is concluded, after a full examination, that performance anxiety in a given case has no physical basis, it does not follow that the psychological factors apparently at work are deep-seated or result from traumatic experiences in early childhood. It is very possible that the problem may result from lack of proper sex education. Some modest counseling may prove to be the solution to the anxiety problem.

For example, gross misconceptions may be taking a toll. Sam, a twenty-five-year-old patient, was highly fearful of entering into any relationship with a woman. There was nothing wrong with Sam physically. During the course of the examination, Sam asked whether anything could be done to increase the size of his penis. His nonerect penis actually measured five inches, well above average. Sam had been avoiding women largely because he feared being ridiculed for a nonexistent physical abnormality.

Mistaken expectations about sex can also underlie performance anxiety. One very undesirable aspect of pornography is that it tends to reinforce the many incorrect ideas about sexual performance first learned in teenage conversations. Exactly what is involved in "satisfying" a woman may be very misunderstood. Although the simultaneous orgasm of both partners is actually not all that frequent, failure for this to occur can result in anxiety in some men. Other men may become very anxious over their failure to perform as well as male actors they have seen in X-rated films. Actually, such films are typically produced over an extended period of time, due to the limited capabilities of the actors. What is seen is really an illusion.

Penile injection therapy, using papaverine, has a role in treating performance anxiety in patients with no identifiable physical problem. Martin, an unmarried psychologist in good health, suffered great anxiety at the beginning of new sexual relationships. Despite counseling, he had not been able to overcome an excessive fear of failure. His solution was an injection prior to the first attempt at sex in a new relationship. The resulting successful performance in each instance gave him the confidence to continue the relationship without resorting to further injections.

Sex therapy plays an important role when psychological problems are deep-seated. More intensive psychotherapy may very well be indicated when the patient's emotional problems are found to include not only anxiety over sexual performance, but also an abnormal level of anxiety about other aspects of behavior.

CHAPTER 11

Getting help —
and what it
will cost

A patient being treated for an impotence problem once was said to have remarked: "Doctor, it's not the performance anxiety that's really bothering me. It's the payment anxiety."

This story, while probably apocryphal, is nevertheless revealing of a very legitimate problem. Treatment does cost money. The costs, moreover, can clearly be a serious consideration to the typical patient, particularly when a penile implant is indicated. Very often, a man requiring an implant is at an age when limited family financial resources must be allocated among a variety of pressing demands. These demands may include the cost of tuition for university-age children, the support of aging parents, the expenses for treating other medical problems, or savings for retirement. The need for treatment may occur at the very time when the patient had hoped to have something left over for such reasonable pleasures of life as international travel, a vacation home, or even frequent meals out. Under the circumstances, it is not uncommon for the patient to feel guilty about spending money on something as "selfish" as personal sexual pleasure.

It is important, therefore, to be aware that the actual out-of-pocket costs may prove to be less than feared. Total treatment costs may also be subject to some degree of control, through careful planning by the patient. Furthermore, the costs should be weighed against the benefits, which are not limited to just the patient's sexual pleasure. After weighing all the factors, this could be one of the best investments that the patient could make for his entire family.

The purpose of this chapter is to provide reasonable estimates of the total overall cost of obtaining help. In most circumstances, this involves the net total cost to the patient after any reimbursements from medical insurance programs. Many patients may also be in the position to reduce the total cost by taking deductions still allowable under current federal and state income tax codes.

Costs shown in this chapter are typical of those prevailing in late 1987 in one large American urban area. Costs, of course, vary throughout the country. Unfortunately, medical costs, in general, have been continually rising for the past several decades, and there is no reason to anticipate this trend will stop. You are cautioned, therefore, to update the information given, and make reasonable allowances for local conditions.

ESTIMATING THE TOTAL COST

Costs for the treatment of male sexual dysfunction logically fall into two general categories. First, there are the charges that will be incurred in diagnosing the problem. Second, there are the expenses that will be incurred in treatment.

Costs of diagnosing the problem

As is the practice of all physicians, urologists specializing in male sexual dysfunction charge for their professional time and any special tests or other procedures that may be required. The number of visits and tests that may be required, of course, depends upon the patient and the problem. As noted in Chapter 6, a reliable diagnosis of an impotence problem can often be achieved in two or three visits. The following is an example of the charges that were incurred by one patient in arriving at a diagnosis of his problem.

Item	Charge
Initial office visit and detailed examination	$ 70
Follow-up visits — two at $30 per visit	60
Blood tests — testosterone and prolactin levels	250
Penile blood flow test	30
Penile snap gauge test	50
Urinalysis — two at $10 each	20
Total billed to patient	$480

The charge shown in the previous example for blood testing may seem excessive compared to the relatively modest charge incurred for routine blood testing in an annual physical examination. The high cost reflects the complex analytical procedures that are performed in the laboratory when determining the hormonal levels. In some instances, the cost for blood testing during an initial visit proves to be somewhat less when a broad spectrum of blood characteristics is not indicated.

In the example shown, the patient's impotence problem was found to be largely due to an abnormally low level of testosterone. The total cost incurred by the patient in reaching an accurate diagnosis is fairly typical for this type of condition.

Total cost for diagnosis, of course, varies depending upon the circumstances. If a corpora cavernosagram, for example, is indicated, a typical charge is $175. Costs can mount when nocturnal penile tumescence monitoring is necessitated. Some insurance companies insist upon this procedure. When this is the case, and the facilities of a hospital sleep lab are used, a charge of $800 per night is not unusual, and the procedure can extend over three nights. When home testing using a portable monitor is acceptable, the cost typically falls in the range of $100 to $150 per night. When the simple snap gauge test is sufficient, the cost, as indicated in the preceding example, is typically about $50.

Costs of treating the problem

Typical charges that are often incurred in the treatment of impotence are shown in the accompanying table. From this information, it should be possible to arrive at a reasonable preliminary estimate of what treatment might cost you, depending on the nature of the problem, and taking into consideration geographical variations in your part of the country.

Treatment, of course, might turn out to cost virtually nothing, should the problem be easily solved by switching to alternative drugs for the control of a high blood pressure problem. The cost for treatment is generally moderate when hormone or drug therapy is indicated. Obviously, penile implants and other treatments that necessitate surgical procedures are considerably more expensive. Where a penile implant is indicated, total costs can vary over a fairly wide range, depending on the type of implant selected by the patient and options as to hospitalization.

REPRESENTATIVE TREATMENT CHARGES[1]

Hormone and Drug Therapy

Item	*Charge*
Regular office visits — per visit	$30 - 35
Office testosterone injection	$10 - 15
Testosterone pellet implant	$250 - 300
Office papaverine injection	$75 - 90
Home papaverine injection	$15 - 20

Treatments Necessitating Surgical Procedures

Item	*Charge*
Penile Implant	
Cost of prosthesis	$4,000
Urologist's surgery fee[2]	$3,000 - 3,250
Anesthesiologist's fee	$350 - 375
Anesthesia supplies	$175 - 200
Use of hospital surgery and recovery facilities	$1,250 - 1,500
Hospital room — per day	$300 - 350
Drugs	$150

Treatments Necessitating Surgical Procedures
(Continued)

Item	*Charge*
Other Surgical Procedures[3]	
Phalloplasty for correction of penile angulation	500
Peyronie's disease plaque removal	600
Penile prosthesis repair	$1,600

[1]*Late 1987*

[2]*Inflatable implant (usually includes office follow-up)*

[3]*Urologist's professional fee*

Hormone and drug therapy

As noted in Chapter 7, patients have several treatment options with testosterone therapy. If the patient chooses to have testosterone injected by the physician during monthly office visits, annual treatment cost would normally be in the $450 to $500 range, including physician's fees and drug cost. The cost will be cut to about half when the patient is willing to inject himself at home. Should the implantation of testosterone pellets under the skin be preferred, the typical cost for the entire procedure, with a sufficient number of pellets to be effective in most patients for about one year, would be about $300.

Determining the annual cost of papaverine injection treatments for impotence is more complicated. There is an initial cost, incurred for the series of office visits during which correct dosage level is determined experimentally, and the patient is carefully trained in proper procedures. The initial cost would include the charge for injections and the normal office visit charge. Subsequently, the patient can inject himself at home, using syringes obtained at the urologist's office which are prefilled with the proper amount of the drug. Alternatively, the patient may fill syringes at home, using a bottle of the drug supplied by the urologist. If the former approach is used, a cost of $15 might be incurred each time sexual activities were desired. In the latter approach, the patient normally incurs a cost of about $100 per bottle. Exactly how long the bottle would last obviously depends on dosage requirement, which can range from 0.1 to 0.4 cubic centimeters per patient, and on the frequency of sexual activities.

Surgical treatments

The first thing to consider in estimating the cost of a penile implant is the selection of a prosthesis. The advantages and disadvantages of the more common devices on the market are discussed in Chapter 8. The more complicated inflatable implants naturally cost the most to purchase and install. A top-of-the-line inflatable prosthesis typically is available for about $4,000. The fee to insert the device typically would be approximately $3,000. In contrast, the costs for obtaining a semirigid prosthesis and for insertion would typically be about one-half of that amount.

A second major factor that determines the total cost of a penile implant is the choice as to where the insertion will take place. Depending upon the patient, there may be a choice between insertion on an inpatient basis at a hospital, insertion on an outpatient basis at a hospital, or insertion on an outpatient basis in a clinical facility. In general, anybody using a hospital's facilities is considered an inpatient, and is charged full price for room and board if an overnight stay is involved. Given average prevailing rates for a semiprivate room, an implant inpatient might incur a charge of about $900 for a three-day hospital stay. Total room charges, however, could be cut to about $100 when the implant procedure is done in a hospital on an outpatient basis. Clinical patients are treated in a physician's office that is equipped with surgical facilities, or at an ambulatory "surgicenter." Implant patients normally avoid all room charges when treated in a clinical facility.

In addition to room charges, there are also potential cost savings to outpatients treated at clinics. Such patients normally avoid hospital charges for surgical and recovery facilities and anesthesia fees and supplies. They are also usually charged at lower rates for drugs.

Given the various options, the overall current cost for a penile implant could range from as low as $7,000 to as high as $14,000. The lower end of the range might apply in the case of a patient requesting a semirigid implant that could be inserted in a clinic and on an outpatient basis. The higher end would apply to a patient requesting an inflatable implant and electing insertion as a hospital inpatient.

Saving money is not the only factor that a patient should consider when reviewing his options as to where insertion of an implant should take place. In making a decision, important factors to consider include the patient's general medical condition, his ability to withstand pain and discomfort, and convenience. Inpatient treatment does offer definite advantages with regard to the control of complications, the minimization of pain, and insuring patient compliance with postoperative instructions. On the other hand, there are many individuals who greatly dislike a hospital environment and would prefer to recuperate in the privacy of their homes.

It is difficult to generalize as to the costs of other surgical procedures. At the low end of the spectrum are the relatively modest fees for the repairing of problems associated with Peyronie's disease. Surgery to remove an arterial blockage, however, constitutes a major medical procedure that typically results in significant charges for surgery and hospitalization.

Sex therapy

Sex therapy is usually billed on an hourly basis, with the charge varying significantly depending upon the academic training, general reputation, and geographical location of the therapist. Medical psychiatrists certified by the American Board of Psychiatry and Neurology typically command higher fees than clinical psychologists with Ph.D.s. Other therapists with lesser credentials usually charge less. Fees charged in major urban areas are usually much higher than those in smaller cities. At present, fees charged by psychiatrists throughout the U.S. average about $75 per "hour." The "hour" is typically fifty minutes. Psychologist fees average about $70 per hour. Fees for other therapists can be as low as $25 per hour.

Intensive traditional psychotherapy can require as many as three sessions per week and possibly extend over a period of years. At the $75 rate charged by psychiatrists, this could result in an annual charge of about $12,000. At one session per week, the charge could add up to about $4,000 per year. Under some circumstances, it may be possible to reduce costs by obtaining treatment through a local mental health center, where there is some adjustment based on ability to pay.

Intensive therapy of the Masters and Johnson type, that takes place over a short time, is usually billed on an overall treatment program basis. The total cost is typically quite expensive, especially when treatment takes place on a residence basis and results in travel and lodging expense in addition to the actual treatment expense.

WHAT WILL INSURANCE PAY?

Insurance company attitudes

It is no secret that the ability to obtain medical services is increasingly dependent on the existence of a cooperative third party that is willing to pick up a major share of the tab. Such third parties include private insurance carriers, union health and welfare organizations, and publicly supported programs such as the Medicare system. Fortunately, most third parties to date have exhibited a reasonably enlightened view toward the coverage of male sexual dysfunction.

Medical insurance is a difficult subject, given the large number of individual insurance carriers, the many different plans that are offered, and the "fine print" characteristics of most insurance policies. Usually, claims submitted in connection with a physician's diagnosis of impotence or other types of dysfunction are approved by the typical claim examiner, unless there is a specific exclusion of this type of claim in the applicable policy. Many policies, however, exclude claims for "routine" visits to physicians' offices or visits that are "not medically necessary." Refusal to reimburse a claim for the diagnosis of an impotence problem, on the grounds that the physician's services are not medically necessary, is unlikely in view of the close linkage between dysfunction and diabetes, arteriosclerosis, and other serious diseases.

Claims for the treatment of impotence that involve hormonal and drug therapy are also usually reimbursed without too much difficulty. Men requiring testosterone supplementation may be subject to a variety of recognized medical problems, in addition to impotence, such as serious loss of physical vigor and muscular atrophy. Insurance companies have also raised little objection to penile injection therapy.

Individuals who have specific coverage in their insurance policies for the treatment of mental and nervous disorders usually do not experience too much difficulty in obtaining reimbursement for at least part of the cost of psychological and sex therapy. Many insurance policies, however, still do not provide adequate coverage in this area, with a $1,000 annual limitation very common. In some cases, the cost per visit and the number of visits to therapists are subject to significant limitations. Carriers are also known to pressure policyholders to utilize the services of therapists who bill at lower hourly rates.

Reimbursement of the cost of a penile implant is a matter of obvious concern. The accompanying table summarizes the current situation. The information shown is, by necessity, general in nature. Plans vary from company to company and are constantly changing.

REPRESENTATIVE INSURANCE COVERAGE
OF PENILE IMPLANT CLAIMS

Plan or Carrier Category	*Typical Coverage*
Blue Cross/Blue Shield	Coverage is generally good. Plans offered under the Blue Cross/Blue Shield name do vary throughout the United States and occasionally change. In some instances, regional groups may exclude dysfunction.
Commercial Group Plans (plans available to employees or members of affinity groups)	Coverage in most plans offered through well-known national insurance carriers is generally very good. Plans occasionally change with minimum prior notices.
Commercial Individual Plans	Coverage is generally good. Many plans, however, are subject to high deductibles. Restrictive waiting periods for eligibility are quite common.

Plan or Carrier Category	*Typical Coverage*
Self-Funded Employer Plans	Fair to good coverage, depending upon company. Exclusion of dysfunction is rare. The professional staffs of in-house company clinics are often important influences in approving coverage.
Health Maintenance Organizations (HMOs)	Coverage is generally only poor to fair. Many HMOs limit or exclude specific types of prostheses, and/or limit reimbursement to a fixed percent of total cost.
Union Health and Welfare Plans	Large unions that operate on a national basis usually offer good coverage. Coverage can be only poor to fair with smaller unions and independent bargaining units. Elective surgery is very often not covered in the contracts of most small unions.
Plans for Federal, State, and Local Government Employees, and the U.S. Postal Service	Coverage varies between individual employee groups, but is generally not generous. Dysfunction is often specifically excluded. A few plans do offer good coverage.

Plan or Carrier Category	*Typical Coverage*
CHAMPUS	Coverage in most existing plans covering retired armed forces personnel and dependents of armed forces personnel is typically very restricted and limited to special situations.
Veterans Administration	Coverage is possible and typically generous when a case can be made that the treatment is necessary for the rehabilitation of a service-connected disability.
Workers' Compensation	State-operated workers' compensation programs usually provide excellent coverage for dysfunction problems that can be demonstrated to have a job-related origin. In most instances, this would mean a physical injury sustained on the job.
Medicare	Coverage of dysfunction is excellent. Claims for dysfunction subject to standard Medicare deductibles.
Medicaid	Coverage may be possible, but only after approval and depending on individual circumstances.

Plan or Carrier Category	Typical Coverage
Automobile and Public Liability Plans	Coverage depends upon the ability of the victim to demonstrate wrongful injury and may involve litigation. Impairment of sexual function is a recognized injury for which compensation can be claimed regardless of the age and marital status of the victim.
Automobile No-Fault Plans	Coverage is generally excellent. States with no-fault laws usually establish caps on allowable medical and surgery fees.

Insurance tips

Insurance companies are typically very happy to receive your premium payments. They are not nearly as enthusiastic when it comes to the payment of claims. In fairness, insurance fraud does exist, and claim examiners must be vigilant in order to protect the public from ever-rising premium levels. Unfortunately, some claim examiners still do not fully recognize the medical necessity of treatment for male sexual dysfunction, and may be inclined to resist reimbursement of claims in this area.

The following are some useful tips in protecting your personal interests in dealing with insurance companies:

- *Fully understand your insurance program* — Read and fully understand the terms and conditions of any existing insurance coverage. If necessary, obtain a complete and detailed description of your coverage. Before making any firm arrangements for treatment, carefully review the "fine print" in your policy. Look especially carefully at sections with titles such as "not covered," "plan does not pay for," "special limitations," and "exclusions and limitations."

- *Be aware of waiting periods* — If changing jobs or retiring, review your new insurance coverage in advance. Be particularly careful of any waiting periods that apply to your new coverage or exclusions that apply to preexisting conditions.

- *Prior approval* — Before committing to any treatment program involving a major expenditure, be sure to obtain prior approval *in writing* from your insurance company. Many insurance companies now insist on prior approval for any type of surgery, and often insist on a second opinion. Failure to obtain prior approval can often result in as much as a 50 percent penalty.

- *Use your physician* — Your physician and his or her professional business staff are a major source of help on insurance matters. Your physician will play a key role in obtaining prior approval from your insurance company, both with respect to communicating your medical history and explaining the importance of the treatment from the standpoint of your physical and mental health and general well-being.

- *Recognize the importance of your treatment* — If you find that you are encountering resistance on the part of your insurance company, it may be necessary for you to be insistent in claiming your coverage. Astute claim examiners are aware that many men subject to dysfunction may feel awkward and defensive and, hence, are at a disadvantage. The best way to deal with this problem is to be fully convinced of the importance of the treatment to your personal well-being and also to remember that, either directly or indirectly, you paid for the insurance coverage.

FINALLY — A POSSIBLE TAX DEDUCTION

Contrary to popular belief, the Tax Reform Act of 1986 did not completely eliminate all tax deductions. As of 1987, persons who itemize deductions on their federal tax return may still take a deduction for all medical and dental expenses allowable under the tax code. The medical and dental deduction beginning in 1987, however, is not worth as much as it once was to the typical taxpayer. For tax years beginning after 1986, the deduction is limited to that part of medical and dental expenses in excess of 7.5 percent of "adjusted gross income." In 1986, the deduction was that part of medical and dental expenses in excess of 5.0 percent of adjusted gross income. Despite this change, there still may be significant savings in federal and state taxes which, of course, serve to reduce the net cost of treatment for sexual dysfunction.

Expenses in connection with the treatment of sexual dysfunction that are usually deductible include:

- The cost of prescription medicine and drugs
- Physicians' professional fees and payments made directly to physicians for tests and drugs
- Payments for tests made directly to medical laboratories
- Psychologist and sex therapist fees
- Hospital costs
- The cost of an implanted penile prosthesis
- Associated transportation expenses

The various costs incurred in the treatment of sexual dysfunction are, of course, grouped with all other medical and dental expenses on the annual tax return. The expense total can include the annual cost for medical, surgical, and hospitalization insurance.

Given the complexity of the tax code, it is usually advisable to seek advice on tax matters from an accountant or other qualified professional. A possible area of concern as to deductibility could be payments made to psychologists or sex therapists. As it should be clear to the readers of this book, such practitioners should be used judiciously in any event. Another gray area where an accountant could be helpful involves expenses incurred in connection with impotence support groups. These expenses are normally minimal. It is possible that some portion may be treated as a charitable contribution.

It is important to recognize that the overall value of any possible tax deduction for the treatment of sexual dysfunction depends on a variety of factors, including the patient's annual taxable income, the additional income of a spouse, the extent of deductions for other medical and dental services, and the amount of insurance coverage. There is no deduction, of course, if deductions are not itemized. In many instances, the new 5.0 percent of adjusted gross income limitation on medical and dental expenses, combined with good insurance coverage, will effectively cancel out the deduction. On the other hand, the deduction could be of importance in the case of a patient with a relatively low adjusted gross income, limited insurance coverage, and significant expenditures for other medical and dental problems. In addition, there may be other favorable consequences for individuals subject to state and local income taxes.

CHAPTER 12

Helping yourself
through prevention

I n most men, loss of potency is associated with increasing age. The reasons are not difficult to understand. Arteriosclerosis is associated with increasing age. Testosterone production peaks in most men in their thirties. Diabetes often does not appear until well into adulthood. As men age, it becomes more likely that some surgical procedure will be required that could have unfortunate consequences with respect to sexual performance. Also, with increasing age, the ravages of alcohol abuse and tobacco gradually take their toll.

The previous chapters deal with the techniques now available to treat dysfunction problems after they have already made their appearance. This chapter provides some basic tips on what you can do to prevent problems or, at least, to delay their appearance.

Men experiencing dysfunction all too often become the marks of quacks and charlatans touting miracle cures. On occasion, some men with perfect sexual function also become victims in the hope of achieving some perceived heroic standard of sexual performance. Impotence fraud has its amusing aspects. The costs, unfortunately, include not only loss of hard-earned cash, but also wasted time and even impairment of health. This chapter provides some basic tips on how to prevent the problems of impotence fraud.

EIGHT TIPS FOR IMPOTENCE PREVENTION

It has been said that life is sometimes unfair. Even the most responsible individual may suffer from dysfunction as a result of an unavoidable accident or perhaps a military service injury. Genetic factors have been identified in many of the physical conditions linked to impotence. Some men have just been dealt a set of bad genes. Nevertheless, most men do have some options.

The tips for preventing impotence are largely the same as those for maintaining good health: proper nutrition, weight control, reasonable exercise, moderate alcohol consumption, avoidance of tobacco and harmful drugs, and life-style control, including control of sexual activities. It is not our intention to preach on these matters, as most people have already been scolded enough. In fact, there is reason to suspect that constant nagging is actually unproductive. Therefore, the discussion accompanying most of the following tips is mainly limited to a brief statement of obvious facts. An exception is the more complicated matter of proper control of your life style.

Tip 1 — Maintain good nutrition.

Most reasonably well-informed individuals are aware of the general rules for good nutrition. These include controlling the consumption of salt and sodium-containing foods, minimizing total fat intake, avoiding foods high in saturated fats and cholesterol, and limiting the intake of refined carbohydrates. The overall implications are a diet that emphasizes fish, chicken, fruits, vegetables, and whole grains at the expense of red meats, certain dairy products, eggs, and junk, fast, and processed foods. Such a diet rarely requires any form of vitamin and mineral supplementation.

Poor diet can result in impotence in three basic ways. First, a diet high in salt and fats can lead to high blood pressure. Unfortunately, as noted, many of the medications used to control hypertension are linked to impotence. Second, a diet high in fats, especially saturated fats and cholesterol, can lead to vascular problems, a major factor underlying impotence. Finally, excessive carbohydrate intake is a factor in diabetes, a major cause of impotence.

Tip 2 — Control your weight.

Good nutrition implies both a properly balanced diet and control of total caloric intake. Obesity contributes directly to both high blood pressure and diabetes. What most people do not know is that there is a natural biochemical conversion of protein to fat, which can take place within the body when caloric intake is excessive. This means that even with a high protein diet a possible buildup of fatty substances can result within the vascular system that also contributes to impotence.

Tip 3 — Get reasonable exercise.

Exercise serves to prevent impotence in several ways. First, a suitable exercise program promotes general cardiovascular fitness. Second, regular exercise lowers blood cholesterol levels. Finally, regular exercise aids considerably in weight control. Sexual activity, incidentally, is a form of exercise, but not one that you can count on for effective weight control. A five-minute sexual interlude for most men might burn up only sixty-five calories. Of course, every bit helps.

Most forms of exercise improve cardiovascular fitness. Exceptions are simple calisthenics, weight lifting, and yoga. There is little benefit from golf when golf carts substitute for walking. For most men over fifty, regular walking and swimming represent the best bet.

Tip 4 — Control alcohol consumption.

The strong link between alcoholism and impotence was emphasized in Chapter 4. Control of alcohol does not imply total prohibition in an individual not prone to alcoholism. An occasional drink by a nonalcoholic under social circumstances is not a cause for any concern. When consumption begins to regularly exceed two drinks per day, there is good reason to bring things under control.

Good control is also a matter of how fast you drink and what you drink. Drinking slowly puts less strain on the liver, where alcohol is metabolized, and thus serves to minimize long-range adverse effects on testosterone and estrogen levels. Diluted drinks help, as you tend to take in alcohol at a slower rate, and will probably drink less in social circumstances.

Tip 5 — Avoid tobacco.

It is difficult to have too much sympathy for any man who is concerned about impotence, but still continues to smoke. The highly addictive nature of tobacco is such, however, that many men and women continue to smoke even after being diagnosed with tobacco-related diseases such as cancer.

The question as to whether secondary tobacco smoke, smoke from the cigarettes of others, can seriously cause adverse consequences, is a controversial matter. It would be best to avoid exposure, although obviously this not always possible. In fact, it is a good idea to attempt to avoid exposure to all airborne pollutants, given their possible cardiovascular consequences.

Tip 6 — Avoid harmful drugs.

The link between impotence and many other controlled substances could be a more compelling reason for some individuals to avoid use than the legal consequences. In the case of legal drugs prescribed by physicians, it is, of course, desirable to avoid use whenever medically possible. The list of drugs linked to impotence in Chapter 5 should be helpful in this connection. It is a good idea to take the initiative in asking about all possible side effects when obtaining a prescription, and not wait for the physician to volunteer this information.

One area where you have some control is with common over-the-counter medications. It is a good idea to avoid most common cold and sleeping remedies, given the possible presence of antihistamines and other chemical entities linked to impotence. Most of these preparations are also of limited effectiveness. When it comes to the relief of cold symptoms, your best bet remains aspirin or acetaminophen.

Tip 7 — Control your life style.

It is conventional wisdom that sexual performance is enhanced by relaxation and the avoidance of stress. While there is some truth to this, it is not always practical. Furthermore, individuals vary greatly in the ways they react to stressful situations.

A letter to the *New York Times* published August 25, 1986, states, "Sexual dysfunction is the first symptom of significant psychopathology in a large percentage of men who are desperately trying to obtain and/or maintain success in the business world." There is a problem with this observation, in that it may give the false impression that impotence is a natural consequence of the stress placed on individuals striving for success. First, there are many highly successful or aspiring men in the business and professional world who continue to perform very well sexually despite crushing day-to-day burdens. Second, there is no hard statistical evidence that business and professional men have a disproportionate incidence of impotence, as compared to men in presumably more bucolic pursuits. Finally, there is considerable evidence that the physical problems associated with impotence — high blood pressure, alcoholism, and so forth — are more common in men at the bottom of the pyramid.

Part of the story could be that it is not so much stress, operating through some mysterious pathway of the mind, that directly causes impotence, but the longer-range consequence of the way men react to stress. If the only way you can cope with stress is with the three-martini lunch, gorging at the table, or chain smoking, the probability increases that a disease such as arteriosclerosis, could, in turn, lead to impotence. If this is the case, a major life-style change involving your job, and probably your income, could represent the only strategy to prevent impotence.

Tip 8 — Control your sexual activities.

The realities of the aging process suggest reasonable adjustments of past sexual patterns. Sexual activities that take place when the chances for failure are greatest obviously can contribute to performance anxiety. One simple adjustment is to plan sexual activities for first thing in the morning. As testosterone levels are highest in men after a good night's sleep, chances of successful sexual performance are the greatest in these circumstances.

In general, it is a good idea to avoid sexual heroics along with conditions not conducive to sexual performance. The age-old institution of the orgy demonstrates that many men in top physical condition can perform in a highly distracting environment. Most men, however, are stretching their luck under such circumstances. In any event, it is quality that counts in sex, as in every other form of human activity.

HOW TO AVOID BEING "TAKEN" — TIPS FOR IMPOTENCE FRAUD PREVENTION

There is nothing new about impotence fraud. There is good reason, however, to suspect that it is becoming increasingly common. Impotent men, since time immemorial, have been easily taken in because of their especially high degree of vulnerability.

Quacks and charlatans often obtain their victims from responses to advertisements placed in sexually oriented magazines or in magazines with highly macho themes. The ads are typically placed toward the rear of the magazines, accompanied by other ads touting preparations purporting to increase penis size, various devices to be used during sex, "swingers" clubs, and bogus hair growth remedies. Another way that victims are found is through direct mail solicitations. The perpetrators are especially adept at obtaining mailing lists containing the names of older men. Porno stores, such as found in the vicinity of Times Square in New York, are another marketing channel.

Quacks with more sophisticated scams, such as pseudoscientific psychotherapy or purported treatments based on the mysteries of the Orient or the occult, sometimes obtain victims through advertisements or through free announcements placed in neighborhood or leisure-time newspapers in large cities. Sometimes, victims are snared through items placed on bulletin boards in health food stores.

The following are a few tips for preventing impotence fraud.

*Tip 1 — Beware of all solicitations that use a blatantly
suggestive sexual theme.*

Solicitations that contain soft-porn pictures or titillating advertising copy deserve to be rejected. Impotence is a medical problem and, while promotional activities are permitted to some extent in the medical field, such activities are limited to the presentation of factual material and generally accepted standards of good taste.

*Tip 2 — Beware of all solicitations that are too good
to be true or that are ridiculous.*

Fraud should be suspected whenever a solicitation offers to provide a medication, service, or some form of information that offers rapid and guaranteed results. As noted in Chapter 7, the only medications now in common use for the treatment of impotence are yohimbine, papaverine, and testosterone. They should only be used under medical supervision. Nevertheless, the African rhinoceros has become an endangered species due to the continuing belief in the Far East that the ground horn of a rhinoceros will improve potency. Young men continue to be taken in Tijuana and other border cities by the hawkers of "Spanish Fly."

Some forms of medication promoted by quacks can be dangerous. One example is chelation therapy, which has been promoted for treatment of hardening of the arteries, as well as for impotence. Men sometimes sniff amyl nitrate and other aromatic substances in the belief that it enhances the orgasm. The real result may be a severe headache or even damage to internal organs.

Penis size nostrums fall under the category of the ridiculous. It is said that "one size fits all." Nevertheless, some men develop performance anxiety over an imagined problem.

Tip 3 — Beware of all solicitations from individuals
    with questionable professional qualifications.

It is a mistake to believe that the medical establishment is the respository of all wisdom. The history of medicine does include many instances of the rejection of ideas later proven to be valid. Outsiders, such as the chemist, Louis Pasteur, have also made major contributions to the medical field. Nevertheless, there is very good reason to be cautious of solicitations made by individuals with credentials well out of the mainstream or with no credentials at all, or of solicitations by misunderstood or rejected would-be geniuses.

A few excerpts from a direct mail solicitation bearing a North Carolina return address sum it all up:

> Close your eyes and imagine the ecstasy of making love to a woman like the one whose picture is enclosed. [The solicitation includes a glossy, three-by-five-inch color photograph of an attractive, suggestively clad woman.]

> If you're not as firm as you were in your teens and 20s — let me tell you about a natural way to regain rock solid potency that works like a miracle.

> After years of frustration, I met an old friend. He told me how his sex life had turned around by following some *very simple instructions.*

> The secrets that my friend revealed to me have been published in a special report: *How To Restore Your Potency.*

> And now for the *good news. How To Restore Your Potency* is yours for only $19.95.

How To Restore Your Potency will do just that — restore
your potency. If it does not, you may return the
report for double your money back.

Thinking that perhaps we had missed something, we
rushed off our $19.95 payment. About a week later, a thirty-
one page soft-cover booklet arrived in the mail. The secret
promised in the advertisement turned out to be "Shiatsu,"
a method of massage, described as "the ancient Oriental
technique for erotic arousal." Shiatsu is said to be widely
practiced in Turkey, Egypt, China, and Japan and obviously
for good reason. Shiatsu will not only restore your potency,
but will cure chronic constipation, skin rash, headaches,
backaches, ulcers, and even heart conditions.

How to perform Shiatsu is described at length in the
booklet, including such valuable details as proper room
temperature, the use of banana, almond, and avocado oils,
and the suggestion that nails should be trimmed very short
to avoid scratching. Among the more fascinating items of
extraneous information provided is the revelation that men
who prefer women with small buttocks generally were
breast fed as infants and do not read sports magazines.
Women with large buttocks, however, are valued by men
who, among other things, are orderly in their everyday
affairs.

Don't say that you weren't warned.

CHAPTER 13

A message
to the partner

S truggling with the burden of male sexual dysfunction is more than just a problem faced by the afflicted man. The impact on you, the partner, can be equally as devastating. Furthermore, you may already suspect that other members of your family unit sense something is very wrong.

With impotence, the female partner and any other members of the household bear the burden of day-to-day living with a deeply troubled man. This is a man who questions his very self-worth. The internal torment comes out in different ways, depending on the man. Perhaps your partner is the type of man who keeps it all to himself. He never talks about the subject and deliberately avoids the tender moments you once so much enjoyed, out of fear that it could lead to still another sexual disappointment. Then again, your partner could be the type who frets incessantly over the problem. He repeatedly attempts intercourse, each time becoming more visibly discouraged.

No matter how he handles the problem, you are increasingly alarmed about certain aspects of his behavior. He always used to be so easy to get along with. Now he seems to snap at you every time you talk to him. His views about almost everything are tinged with bitterness. He is drinking much more heavily and after many years of abstinence, has resumed smoking. He is having problems on the job. He is obviously deeply depressed and has said several times recently that life is hardly worth living.

You, of course, have your own sexual needs, but you are afraid to say anything. Perhaps you consider your sexual drive relatively modest and are willing to accept lack of fulfillment. Nevertheless, the problem has filled you with self-doubts and perhaps even suspicions. Maybe it is something that you have or have not done. Maybe he no longer considers your physical appearance attractive. Maybe he no longer considers you interesting to be with. Perhaps his problem has been caused by your lack of enthusiasm or imagination when you make love. Then again, perhaps the real problem is that your partner is having an affair, leaving him too worn out for sex with you at home.

Perhaps you are of the age to have children and want to do so. How can this ever be possible given your partner's problem? Maybe having children is not such a good idea, anyway, given the way things have been going.

Unfortunately, there are no miracle solutions. The following, however, are a few tips that should be helpful:

Tip 1 — Tell your partner that you fully realize a serious problem exists.

When an impotence episode occurs, it is a very common pattern for women to attempt to console their partners with statements such as, "It's not important," or "It doesn't matter." Such words, while sincere and loving in intent, are often very counterproductive. Despite what is being said, the man knows that the problem really does matter, and not only to himself.

It is far better to tell your partner that you know there is a serious problem that very much matters to both of you. Emphasize to your partner that you know the problem is not due to any failing on his part. Make it clear that you know there are effective solutions. Finally, tell him that this is something that both of you are going to work out together.

> *Tip 2 — Encourage your partner to perform the personal evaluation outlined in Chapter 5.*

The personal evaluation outlined in Chapter 5 should help you decide whether the problem could be just temporary in nature or something that requires immediate professional attention. Assist your partner whenever possible in making the evaluation. Make a game that both of you can play out of the simple physical tests given in the chapter. A little humor in the situation, even gallows humor, should help both of you. Moreover, you may find that just the fact you are doing something together will make both of you feel much better.

> *Tip 3 — If indicated, encourage your partner to seek prompt professional attention.*

If the personal evaluation suggests the problem is more than temporary, encourage your partner to immediately seek professional attention. Be especially insistent whenever there is reason to suspect that the impotence problem could be the result of a serious underlying physical problem, such as diabetes. It is also important to let your partner know that the logical way to deal with impotence is to first investigate the possibility of a physical cause. Encourage him to review the material on where to get help in Chapter 6.

> *Tip 4 — Become personally familiar with the causes of impotence, or any other dysfunction problem that your partner may be experiencing.*

While there is no need to become an expert on the subject, it will be potentially very helpful for both of you if you become familiar with the various conditions that can underlie impotence. It can be surprisingly comforting to know that impotence can often have a physical, rather than a psychological, cause. This helps to alleviate any guilt feelings that you or your partner may be experiencing. It also makes you an active partner in the solution of the problem.

> *Tip 5 — Become personally familiar with treatment*
> *methods.*

The more you know about treatment methods, the better position you will be in to assist your partner whenever an important decision as to treatment is required. It is particularly important that you share all decisions regarding a possible penile implant. Also, the more familiar you become with treatment methods, the more helpful you will be to your partner during the actual treatment program.

> *Tip 6 — Investigate alternative sexual techniques.*

Investigate possible ways for you and your partner to achieve mutual sexual satisfaction that do not require full vaginal penetration. It is important to let your partner understand that you do not consider this a substitute for the "real thing," but rather something you can do temporarily while the two of you work together to overcome the impotence problem.

> *Tip 7 — Don't give up should you want to have*
> *children.*

If having children is a factor, it is important that you personally recognize that as long as your partner can ejaculate, you can have children. The process would not be much different than would be the case with artificial insemination, and the baby will be just as precious. Be sure that your partner is aware of these facts.

Tip 8 — *Consider joining a support group with your partner.*

Participation in an impotence support group can prove to be very helpful. Such groups will provide you with valuable information relevant to your problem. Contact with persons with similar problems could prove comforting, as you learn that your problems are not unique and that others have achieved effective solutions.

Workable treatments now exist for male sexual dysfunction. The treatments, of course, are not perfect. After all, there is still no way to repair destroyed nerves or to flush accumulated plaque out of arteries. Available techniques, such as the implant, however, have been found to be very effective.

It is certain that great strides in treatment will occur over the next few years. Remember that only little more than a decade ago, there was very little hope for many patients. Even true psychological impotence can be expected to yield to convenient and economical treatment in the future.

Finally, be aware that solving a male sexual dysfunction problem is not a cure-all for a badly flawed relationship. Working together with your partner to solve the problem, however, can actually strengthen a basically sound relationship. That is what Susan and Jesse, whom you met at the beginning of this book, found out.

Index